Heal Without Medicine

L. B. Coles, MD

Edited by Pete Johnson

Heal Without
Medicine

Edited by Paul Johnson

Heal Without Medicine

L. B. COLES, M.D

CONTENTS

PREFACE

THIS work has been written during irregular and interrupted intervals, which have occurred amidst the pressure of other cares, and has passed through but one manuscript to the press; yet the ideas contained in it are the result of many years' experience, observation, and study; not particularly the study of books and others' theories, but the study of natural law, and the philosophy of facts. And although its leading motto is "Health without Medicine," yet it is not expected that no medicines are ever needed; it is sometimes necessary to take medicine to remove disease — assist nature to throw off her encumbrances, and restore herself to health and strength. Yet whoever will obey nature's laws, will, comparatively speaking, have health without the aid of medicine. Medicines should be used only as unavoidables; they should only be resorted to when the remedy may not be worse than the disease, as a choice between two evils, both of which should be avoided as far as possible.

This manual is not intended particularly for the eye of the medical man, but for the mass of the people. And although the author may be considered ultra by some, on the subject of animal food, yet it is most, sincerely to be hoped that no one will allow himself to imbibe a prejudice against the rest of the work, because he cannot consent to this doctrine; for, let it be remembered, that it is said in the introduction of this topic, that no strenuousness is intended on the subject, but that it is better that every one judge candidly on the matter for himself. While, therefore, the writer would urge — not for himself, but for the good of the community — with all earnestness and solicitude, a serious attention to, and regard for, his views and suggestions on every other topic contained in this work, yet, with all modesty, would he retire from any controversy with those who cannot relinquish the use of meat. He is content with stating what he believes to be the facts in the case, and would leave the decision of the matter entirely with those who may think or act differently.

INTRODUCTION

THERE is scarcely any subject so universally neglected as a knowledge of the laws of health and life. We naturally love to be well, and dread to be sick; yet take little or no pains to economize our health or to ward off disease. We indulge our appetites and inclinations in violation of the laws of health, until we are overtaken with the penalty which the Great Author of our being has affixed to them, in the form of disease, and then, perhaps, charge the result to Divine Providence.

It may, with propriety, be said, that nine cases out of ten, if not ninety-nine out of a hundred, of the ailments which annoy mankind, especially those of a chronic character, might with ease be avoided. We might as well be enjoying health, as a general thing, as to be groaning under pains and diseases. Though we might not be able to repel measles, small-pox, scarlet fever, and many other contagious or epidemic diseases, yet nearly all chronic diseases, and a very large proportion of those which are acute, might be prevented; and even those which could not be avoided, — for instance, that fearful malady, the small-pox, — by habitual obedience to law, would be made of much milder form.

Very little is known by the people at large on this subject, and what is known is very lightly appreciated. Scarcely any subject can be presented to the community in which they take so little interest, as that which immediately concerns their health, until they are overtaken with disease.

And scarcely any subject can be brought forward which is more offensive than this, especially to those who love their appetites more than they do their health.

These few pages are intended for those who are willing to know what course is best in order to retain or to regain a healthy constitution — for those who have more regard for their own ultimate good than for their present gratification — for those who prefer the right way to that which fosters unlawful indulgence.

It is not only a matter of expediency that we obey law in this respect, but a matter of right. The laws which govern our constitutions are the laws of the Creator; and to their violation he has affixed a penalty, which must sooner or later he met. And it is as truly a sin to violate one of these laws, as it is to violate one of the ten commandments. Most people seem to think that they have an undoubted right to do to and with their own bodies as they please; forgetting that God will hold them under obligation to obey physical as well as moral law, and that every infringement of that law will meet with its appropriate reward.

L. B. C.

THE DIGESTIVE ORGANS

THERE is no part of the human system which has such controlling influence over the whole body, as respects health or disease, as the Digestive Organs. Any derangement in these, especially the stomach, calls up a sympathy of action from the whole animal economy. Nearly all the morbid actions found in the general system are produced from causes first operating on the stomach. Hence, keeping the digestive system in a healthy state, secures, as a general rule, a healthy action in every other part of the physical organization. Therefore, to know something of the anatomy and physiology of the digestive organs, together with the laws of digestion, seems indispensable for every individual who would know how to take care of his health.

By the term digestive organs, are intended the Mouth, Stomach, Liver and Bowels, including the whole alimentary canal, commencing with the mouth and terminating with the extremity of the bowels. Extending through the whole length of this canal is a lining membrane, called mucous membrane, continuous throughout, from the lips to the opposite extremity. This membrane is filled, throughout its whole distance, with minute blood-vessels, and in some parts abundantly supplied with fine filaments of nerves. This membrane has important functions to perform in the process of digestion. It is a membrane of much delicacy of structure and sympathy. Its healthy action is easily deranged, and when deranged in one part, becomes, by sympathy, deranged in every part.

THE MOUTH

The mouth, with its teeth and glands, commences the digestive process. The teeth are to masticate the food. The salivary glands give important aid, too, in digestion. There are three pairs of glands which pour the fluid which they secrete into the mouth. This fluid is called saliva. The effort of chewing food excites these glands and promotes the secretion of saliva, which is essential to the healthy digestive process.

THE STOMACH

The stomach is the most important organ of digestion. It has three coats; that which has most to do with digestion is the mucous coat, which lines it. This coat is supposed to furnish by its glands what is called gastric juice; which is the principal agent of digestion in the stomach.

The stomach is abundantly supplied with nerves, and holds a very powerful sway over the whole nervous system; so that when the stomach is under the influence of disease, either acute or chronic, the whole system is immediately in a state of suffering. To secure, then, a healthy system, the stomach must be kept in health.

THE LIVER

The liver has to do with digestion. This organ furnishes the bile. It is the largest gland in the body. Its office seems to be to gather from and carry out of the system substances which, if retained, might prove hurtful. When the liver is inactive, we have what is called jaundice; the liver failing to take up from the system that substance which forms the bile. When this is the case, a yellow substance is found diffused throughout the whole body; the white of the eyes, and sometimes the surface of the whole body, exhibit a yellow tinge.

The bile, when properly secreted and discharged, meets the contents of the stomach as discharged into that part of the bowels nearest the stomach, and is there supposed to assist in the process of separating the nutritious part of that contents from the refuse which is to pass off by the bowels; but its more important office, doubtless, is to aid the passage of the refuse, or the feces, by evacuation. The bile seems to be nature's appropriate stimulus to the bowels; without which costiveness and other irregularities are likely to ensue.

THE BOWELS

The bowels contain the absorbent vessels, which take up the nutritious part of food and carry it into the circulation of the blood for the support of the system. They also convey the refuse part of food out of the body.

THE DIGESTIVE PROCESS

MASTICATION

Mastication, or chewing, is the first step in the process of digestion. When food is taken, it should be thoroughly masticated before it is suffered to pass into the stomach. Without chewing, the food is too coarse and gross for the stomach; and is unprepared for the action of the gastric juice. Besides this, the action of chewing causes the food to be mixed with the saliva; which is an important item in the preparation of it for the action of the stomach and its juice. The food should therefore be broker. up into a fine mass and well moistened with saliva. In order to accomplish this end, it is highly necessary that food should be taken with sufficient moderation to give time for the process of mastication and the discharge of saliva from the glands of the mouth. Eating fast, or even talking while chewing, besides its incongruity with politeness and good breeding, is directly at war with thorough mastication.

Many persons seem to think that hurrying their meals to save time is economy; their business drives them, and they drive their time of meals into the smallest possible compass. This is miserable economy; for when they hurry clown their food, half chewed and half moistened with saliva, it deranges the process of digestion throughout; and, as a consequence, the food not only sets bad on the stomach, and in time causes dyspepsia, but it fails to accomplish the sole object of taking it

— the nourishment of the body. In order to derive nourishment from food, it must be well digested; hence it must be well masticated. When, therefore, we hurry our eating, we hasten our steps on the wrong road. Time curtailed in eating, is worse than hiring money at three per cent. a month. If we cannot spare time to eat, we had better not eat at all. This idea cannot be too deeply impressed: thousands, by this kind of careless, reckless eating, have found themselves the victims of dyspepsia, and all its attendant train of evils. The digestive organs may bear the abuse awhile without giving many signs of trouble; but the penalty of that broken law must, sooner or later, come; and it may come in the form of a broken constitution.

CHYMIFACTION

Chymifaction, or the transformation of food into chyme, is the next important step in the process of digestion. The food, after mastication, passes into the stomach: here it is formed into a homogeneous mass, partly fluid and partly solid, which is called chyme. What is the exact philosophy of this process has been a matter of some discussion, into which it is not necessary now to enter; nor is it yet satisfactorily settled, so as to admit of any definite instruction being given.

The theory which is now generally received respecting the manner in which the stomach acts upon food, is, that the gastric juice possesses a solvent power by which the food becomes reduced to a uniform mass. The solvent power of the gastric juice is very great in healthy, vigorous stomachs; but varies in strength according to the energy of that organ.

The solvent power of the gastric juice is evidently

controlled by the vital principle, or principle of life. While the gastric juice of a healthy stomach acts vigorously upon the hardest kind of food, yet sometimes, when it comes into contact with anything possessed of the principle of life, its power is stayed. Worms, while living, are not affected by it; but when destroyed, are often digested.

The gastric juice possesses the property also of coagulating liquid albuminous substances. The stomach of the calf is used for this purpose by the dairy women, in making cheese. When the infant throws up its milk because the stomach is too full, that milk will be more or less curdled; and instead of considering this curdling an indication of disease, it should be considered a symptom of a healthy stomach.

The time ordinarily occupied in the process of chymifaction, when food has been properly masticated, has been ascertained to be FOUR OK FIVE HOURS. The first hour of this period is occupied in the process of intermixing the food, after it enters the stomach, with the gastric juice. After this is accomplished, an alternation of contraction and expansion of the stomach, or a kind of churning motion, takes place, and continues till the whole mass is converted into chyme, and is conveyed to the first intestine or duodenum, to undergo another change.

CHYLIFACTION

Chylifaction, or the formation of chyle, is the next great step in the process of digestion. This takes place in the duodenum. The chyme from the stomach is let into this intestine little by little. A valve at the lower opening or outlet of the stomach prevents it from passing any faster than it can be disposed of in the formation of chyle. This fluid is a thin milky liquid extracted from the chyme, and then taken up by absorbent vessels, called lacteals.

The chyme passes slowly through the duodenum; and in doing so, becomes mixed with another fluid furnished from the pancreas or sweet-bread, and the bile from the liver. Pass ing thus slowly through this large intestine, ample time is given for the lacteals to take up all that is valuable to be carried into the circulation for the nourishment and support of the system. This chyle, taken up by the lacteals, is directly converted into blood; and in many of its characteristics it very closely resembles blood. The process by which this conversion is carried on, is called absorption. That class of absorbent vessels called lacteals are not only found in the first intestine, or duodenum, but are distributed along the small intestines, for the purpose, as before stated, of conducting the chyle in its appropriate course for the formation of blood.

EVACUATION

Evacuation, or the discharge of the refuse part of food through the bowels, is another, and the last step in the process of digestion. This part of the subject has a very important bearing upon the condition of health. It is impossible for any one to enjoy good health while this office of the bowels is imperfectly performed.

If the bowels are relaxed and irritable, the food is borne along too soon and too rapidly: this causes the process of chylifaction to be imperfect: the chyle is imperfectly formed, and the lacteals have not sufficient time to absorb it from the mass. This prevents the food from nourishing the system. Hence, those who suffer from chronic diarrhea may eat largely, and yet grow weaker and weaker; their food does not nourish them; the nutritious part of it passes off through the bowels instead of being taken into the blood.

If the bowels, on the other hand, are constipated, the consequences are no less unhappy. No one can possibly be well with costive bowels. The free and easy action of the bowels is as truly essential to health, as the free circulation of the blood. When the bowels are sluggish, the process of absorption of the chyle is retarded, and what chyle is absorbed is less pure and healthy; so the quality of the blood is impaired.

Besides the evils already mentioned, a costive state of bowels often causes a pressure of blood on the brain; also derangement of the nervous system — excitability of the nerves; nervous headache; depression of spirits; and a long catalogue of sufferings, too numerous for detail. Habitual costiveness impairs the tone of the stomach, and prevents its healthy action. Piles, also, with various degrees of severity, are often caused, directly or indirectly, by constipated bowels.

The causes of costiveness are various; and to point them out in detail would be perhaps a fruitless toil. But there is one cause, and a very common one, which claims attention here: it is the habit of inattention to, and neglect of the natural promptings of the bowels to evacuate themselves. Thousands on thousands, especially females, by a habit of checking the natural inclinations of the bowels to throw off their contents, have brought upon themselves a habitual costiveness, which, in time, has cost them immense suffering and wretchedness.

No one should ever hold his bowels in check if it be possible to avoid it. It can be readily perceived that doing this would tend to diminish the natural effort of the bowels, and to collect their contents into a solid mass. Then the exertion required to empty the bowels, or the physic taken to aid and make effectual that exertion, tends also to increase the difficulty.

A habit of costiveness should always be removed if possible; and the best way of doing this is by a course of discipline. Those articles of food should be selected which have an influence to keep the bowels open. Bread made of flour has a tendency to constipate them. But brown bread, and bread made of wheat meal, have a tendency to open them; also molasses taken with food has an additional tendency. Fruits and greens, if the stomach can bear them, are adapted to relieve costiveness.

The influence of the mind should also be brought to bear upon this difficulty. The operation of the mind on the physical system is always great, especially in chronic complaints. A person with costive bowels should have a mental determination to have a natural evacuation of the bowels at some regular hour in the morning; just after breakfast should be preferred. By a mental calculation — by bearing the subject in mind — by thinking and desiring — by intending to have the bowels move about that hour, very much may be done by way of facilitating such a result.

But if, instead of attending to a favorable diet, and of thinking on the subject at the proper time, we treat the difficulty with medicines alone, we do harm rather than good; for the more alternatives we take, the more we increase the trouble. The physic only overcomes the constipation for the time, and afterwards leaves the bowels in a more torpid state. Still, rather than endure the consequences of costiveness, it is better to take alternatives, in conjunction with other means, until the difficulty can be overcome. When alternatives are used in conjunction with discipline, they should be of the mildest kind. No proper pains should be spared in overcoming this derangement of nature, till a habitual movement of the bowels, once in twenty-four hours, is secured.

DIETETIC RULES

Time for eating has claims for attention. If persons intend to have health, their meals should be regularly timed and distanced. There is much importance to be attached to the kind of food which we allow ourselves to take; but the time of taking food, together with the proper intervals between meals, has a much more important bearing on our health. Therefore, as just stated, meals should be regularly divided and distanced. A good common rule for the time of meals for the laboring classes, is, breakfast at seven o'clock, dinner at one, and' supper at seven. But at different seasons of the year, and with different classes and occupations in society, the time of meals varies.

But whatever hours may be selected as most convenient for meals, they should be uniform; and for this reason — at the hour when the stomach is accustomed to receive food, the appetite is sharper generally, and the gastric juices more copious, than they are immediately before or after that time. If food be taken before the accustomed hour, the stomach is, as it were, taken by surprise, and is not found in perfect readiness to receive it; if the meal is delayed beyond the accustomed time, common experience teaches that the appetite is liable to lose its sharpness; there is, for a while, less inclination to take food. The objection, however, against delaying a meal beyond the usual time, is very small compared with the objections against eating too soon; because when a meal or luncheon is taken soon after a previous one, the stomach has not had sufficient time to go through with the digestive process, and to recruit its energies for another effort. But when a meal is delayed longer than usual, though the appetite may lose its sharpness for a short time, yet it will return again; and the digestive power of the stomach will not have been impaired, unless the period of abstinence should be of long continuance.

In the arrangement of regular meals, regard should be had to the hour of rest at night. Ten o'clock, as will hereafter be considered, is a favorable hour for retirement; and no food should be previously taken in all ordinary cases within the space of two or three hours. If food be taken too near the time of sleep, so as to leave no chance for the more active parts of the digestive process to be performed, there will be found generally a dull, heavy pain in the head on the following morning, with diminished appetite. The food has laid comparatively undigested through the night; because when we sleep, the whole system is in a quiescent state; the nerves which are called into action in the process of digestion, are, during healthy sleep, inactive. A late supper generally occasions deranged and disturbed sleep; there is an effort on the part of the nerves to he quiet, while the burdened stomach makes an effort to call them into action; and between these two contending efforts, there is disturbance — a sort of gastric riot — during the whole night. This disturbance has sometimes terminated in a fit of apoplexy and in death.

TINE FOR DIGESTING

Time for digesting what is eaten, demands of every one who values health, a most serious consideration. Ignorance on this topic, and inattention to its importance even when understood, have involved thousands and millions in untold suffering and premature death. If it were possible so to impress the mind of community on this subject, that they would obey nature's laws, or rather the laws which the Great Author of nature has given to our digestive systems, we should sec a very obvious change taking place in the standard of general health. The larger portion of people have no rules for eating, but to eat, as they say, "when they are hungry;" having no regard to the time of eating, or to time for digesting; but like the short-fed beasts, take a little here and there, whenever and wherever they can get it. They think their own

stomachs are a sufficient guide, in spite of facts and philosophy. Therefore, they eat whenever they take a notion. Their stomachs would perhaps guide them in the right way if a morbid action of those organs had never been induced by previous irregularities.

Three meals a day are sufficient for all classes of persons, under all circumstances, and of all ages. For persons having weak stomachs, and many persons of sedentary habits, two meals a day, rightly distanced, might be preferable. But no individual, whatever may be his age, his occupation, or his health, should take solid food more than three times in one day. No person can do more than this without transgressing nature's laws. The reasons for this rule will soon be given.

An argument against taking food at regular intervals is often attempted from the fact that many dumb animals have no regular times of eating; and it is urged that these animals have no other guide than the dictates of nature. In answer to this, it may be said, that the habits of dumb beasts, since the introduction of sin into the world, under the weight of which "the whole creation," or rather, as the original signifies, EVERY CREATURE, "groaneth, being burdened," are not always in exact accordance with nature's rules. For instance, cattle are put into a lean pasture; and they are unable to gather a full meal at once; they are obliged, perhaps, to graze all day long to obtain sufficient subsistence. In such cases, to allow intervals between meals, would be to undergo gradual starvation. But put dumb animals into full feed, and what do they do? They deliberately eat a full meal, and then cease eating till that meal is fully digested. Hence, the testimony taken from this source, when we make a fair test, is unequivocally and uniformly in favor of eating at intervals sufficient for digestion.

Eating at intervals sufficiently long to allow the full digestion of a meal before another is taken, is as truly essential to the good constitution and health of beasts, as of human beings. The time was, even within the limits of fifteen or twenty years, when it was customary, on driving a horse on the road, to feed him about every ten miles. This was enough to kill the poor animal; he had no time to digest his food and derive nourishment from it; and it is well that such a system has been abandoned; and it would be better still, if intelligent beings would adopt a similar rule of diet for themselves, and those under their care. Those who drive horses for pleasure-riding or in teaming, at this day, having proved the folly of the old system, feed regularly three times a day. Under this method, the animals eat, on the whole, less in quantity, are found in better order, and endure much more; and why? because they derive, by obedience to nature's law, more nourishment from the same food, and do not break down the digestive organs by oppressing them with too oft-repeated meals, And when individuals live as they list, and eat when they please, in disregard of right rules of diet, they commit a crime against nature. They pin against God, by treating with contempt his laws; they sin against their own bodies, by committing gradual suicide; and the penalty of those violated laws must be met — there is no escape; the punishment will, in some way, sooner or later come. nature's own God will and must take this matter in hand, and sustain the validity of his own laws.

Now for the whys and wherefores of these directions. In the first place, food must be thoroughly masticated; this requires about HALF AN HOUR; especially at dinner, which is, generally and properly, the principal meal for the day. Inattention to and curtailment of time necessary for mastication, is a violation of physical law at the very outset of the digestive process; and one which, more or less, deranges all the other steps. In the second place, when food is lodged in the stomach, it requires ordinarily about FOUR HOURS for this organ to perform its work, before the entire meal is disposed of and carried into the duodenum, or first intestine. Here are, then, at least four hours and a half required for the process thus far; and probably five hours are more often needed, than a period short of four and a half. Then, after this, there remains the process of chylifaction to be finished.

Therefore, no two meals or luncheons should be allowed to come nearer to each other than a distance of at least FIVE HOURS. Because, as any one can see, there is a regular routine of steps, in the process of digestion, to be gone through with in this space of five hours. And if a second meal or lunch be taken short of that period, it produces confusion; the process with the first meal is interrupted; the organs are obliged to stop their course and begin a new process with the second meal: there will be probably a struggle between the two processes, and both be imperfectly performed. By this course, the organs are weakened, and the amount of nutrition from a given quantity of food is much less. To illustrate this method of proceeding and its effects, suppose an omnibus, running between Boston and Cambridge, should set out from Brattle-street with passengers, and after passing half way to Cambridge, the driver should recollect that there are a number more passengers whom he had forgotten; but instead of finishing his present route, and taking those left behind at the next regular trip, he wheels about, brings his load back, takes in the rest, and again proceeds. Precisely analogous to this, is the course which multitudes take in respect to their eating; one meal is half digested, and another is crowded upon it. The organs are kept continually at work, without systematic order, and without chance to rest and recruit their energies.

The good effects of regular and simple diet may be seen by visiting our prisons. There the inmates are generally in possession of good health, notwithstanding their confinement and close air. Some have gone there greatly afflicted with dyspepsia, but have obtained a complete cure, and become robust; and this at the time there must unavoidably have been a great and constant mental oppression. This is incontrovertible testimony in favor of plain and regular living.

Besides the positive injury done to the digestive organs themselves, by eating too often, and, by injury to those organs, a sympathetic injury to the whole system, there is a sort of negative injury done to the entire system by the interruption of the process of nutrition. After breakfast has been taken, let a lunch be eaten about eleven o'clock, and the process of chylifaction and nutrition is broken up, by the digestive energies being attracted too soon to the work of disposing of the eleven o'clock lunch; and so on in the same manner so long as meals and lunches succeed each other without giving at least five hours space for digestion. Hence, the system receives less nourishment from about twice the quantity of food per day, than it would receive under a regular, systematic diet, with a regular quantity.

It is argued by some that the inclination to eat is a proper guide to the time and frequency of eating. But this is no rule at all; if we eat ten times a day habitually, the stomach is obliged to undergo such a change in its action, that we shall think we are hungry as many times. There comes up a disordered action of the stomach, and a morbid appetite ensues. What sort of a guide is a man's inclination to eat who is just merging from the prostrating power of a typhus fever? And why is it that those who are always eating are always hungry; while those who live on three meals a day are not inclined to eat till the regular meal-time comes?

But why contend against facts established by the researches of learned physiologists? They have given us the time required for digestion; we know that this being correctly ascertained, we cannot interrupt that process without detriment. And who is willing to sacrifice justice to himself, and to the Author of his being, for the paltry gratification of a moment? Thousands do it; but it seems too uncharitable to suppose they would do it with their eyes open; though it is to be feared too many are willingly blind.

Whoever knows no law hut the fearful dictates of carnal appetites, is like a ship, driven by fierce winds coastward, without anchor. If we would do right — if we would act upon principle — we must obey every righteous law. That is a safe and prosperous government where obedience to law is sustained; that is a well regulated physical system whose physical law is obeyed. But how sadly this law is trampled under foot. How many there are who reverse one of the best rules of life: while all should EAT TO LIVE, they, impiously and wantonly, LIVE TO EAT. In this way, they destroy the very foundation of all true enjoyment from temporal sources, and prejudice the prospect for the future life. The old heathen adage, "Let us eat and drink, for to-morrow we die," is the sum and substance of their theology — they know no God but their belly.

Time for exercise has an important connection with digestion, and is indispensable to health. It is important to the healthy state of body and mind. Bodily health cannot be secured without doe attention to exercise. Persons of sedentary habits, especially, should give particular attention to this subject. Persons of active or laborious habits can make their business subserve the purpose of exercise; while those whose daily task requires little physical exertion, need some other exercise. By such, let this part of the subject be particularly heeded. To illustrate what is meant, take the case of the shoemaker: his business chains him to the bench; it gives him insufficient bodily exercise; he is too much confined.

The shoemaker, then, or the man of similar occupation, should endeavor to have a garden to cultivate, if in the country, because this is one of the very best kinds of employment for exercise; it affords physical motion and exertion: it gives amusement to the mind, and it secures healthful influences from the earth. If this means cannot be secured, then resort should be had to cutting wood, or some other useful exertion; if this cannot be obtained, then he must resort to some artificial exercise; at all events, some kind of brisk and smart exercise should be had early in the morning before breakfast. This gives activity and energy to the body, greatly invigorates the appetite, and exhilarates the mind. After breakfast, he can go to his bench if he please; but he should never put himself to hard work short of about one hour after taking his meal. He may do light work, but should never put himself to severe exertion in any way for about one hour. This rule applies, as also the previous one, to all sedentary habits. It also applies to every meal. In every case of a similar kind, where exercise is taken for recreation, it should be immediately before each meal, and not immediately after it. And as dinner is generally the heaviest meal, one full hour at least should be allowed after finishing it, for the first step towards digestion, i.e., the mixing of the food with the gastric juice.

Now for a reason for this rule; let the dinner be taken for an illustration: why should we rest from much exertion after taking our dinner? And this rule applies with equal force to all classes of persons and all kinds of business; the reason is this: when a meal is to be digested, or, more properly, while the food is being broken up by the gastric juice, which process occupies in the case of a dinner full one hour, the nervous energies of the whole system are drawn into sympathy with the stomach, and made tributary to this part of the digestive process; their aid is needed: this is a law which the Author of nature has established, and it should be obeyed; i.e., nothing should be allowed to interrupt this natural arrangement. But if we allow ourselves to make much bodily or mental exertion during the hour mentioned, we distract this arrangement; because when bodily exertion is made, the nervous energies are required and drawn in that direction, in aid of the muscular powers; or if the mind is made to labor, then the nervous energies are called in that direction. Hence, when body or mind is taxed considerably immediately after eating, the process of digestion is much disturbed and interrupted.

Everybody's experience corroborates the truthfulness of this theory. We know that after a full meal, especially a dinner, there is a disinclination to much bodily action or mental effort; so strong is the draft upon the nervous energy, or nervous fluid, or animal electricity, whichever it may be called, that it is with difficulty we can call it in any other direction. Therefore, to make much exertion of body or mind immediately after a meal, is to violate a law of the animal economy. To attempt hard work, or study, within one hour after eating, will induce in any one, except the most vigorous system, with a cast-iron stomach, derangement in the functions of the digestive organs; the food will not digest so well, and the system will not be as well nourished from the same quantity of food. Hence, the whole system is impaired, its vigor and durability are diminished, and life is shortened.

It is in vain that we contend that nature has no rules — the Maker of these bodies no laws — violated law no penalty. It is worse than idle to say, here are A, B, and C, — they have lived to a great age — have been robust, and have never observed these rules. The general rule is one thing, and the exceptions make another. These instances appear to be the exceptions to a general rule. But are they really and in all respects exceptions? Because some who have kept their bodies and souls in a gradual steeping of alcoholic liquor have been apparently robust, and have lived to old age, is it proved that alcohol has never done them injury? But while one has lived a long life in violation of law with seeming impunity, a hundred and one, especially of those who have followed sedentary habits, literary men in particular, have gradually ruined their constitutions. Whoever has intelligence enough to know that nature has laws, is in duty bound to obey them, and not run the hazard of laying temptations for disease. And whoever will take the safe side of this matter, will always find it for his good. Even the farmer, in the most driving season of the year, will find obedience to law to be for his interest. Let him conform — and his men with him — to the old maxim, "after dinner sit awhile," even one hour, or, what might be better, instead of sitting idle, let all hands do some light matter such as tinkering and preparing tools, and he will find, in the long run, more work accomplished, with less expenditure of strength.

After exercising very lightly for one hour after eating, then let them begin to increase their amount of labor, and keep themselves pound down to work until the time of another meal. This light exercise, immediately after eating, if it be something artificial, i.e., got up simply for exercise, should not only be light, so as not to require real muscular exertion, but it should be something that is adapted to amuse and exhilarate the mind. The state of the mind has much to do with the health of the body, and especially the healthy and free action of the digestive organs. Hence, it is exceedingly important, in all efforts at exercise, that the mind be interested in whatever the hands undertake. Anything that is a piece of drudgery to the imagination, would be of little service to the body.

The fact that the nervous energies are attracted in the direction of the digestive process immediately after a meal, which renders any considerable physical or mental exertion at that time particularly burdensome, is proved true in the conduct of dumb animals. When the ox or the horse has grazed a full meal, he immediately becomes indisposed for exertion or activity. And the same rule should be observed in regard to his labor, that has been recommended for human beings; he should never be forced into hard labor short of one hour after he has eaten his meal. The ferocious animals, when they have taken a full meal, lose for a time their fierceness, and are comparatively harmless. And so it is with man; if it be necessary to ask a favor of a morose or tigerish man, seek an interview immediately after dinner; if a charity is to be solicited from a creature who carries a miser's soul within his encasement of flesh, see him immediately after dinner, At any other time than after a full meal, they would resist, and succeed, probably, in warding off every motive; but while the nervous energies are taxed with the digestive effort, they cannot rouse themselves so well to meet the emergency; they will rather grant the favor asked, than annoy themselves with the effort necessary to repel the invader.

TIME FOE LABOR

Time for labor, taken in its relation to the time of taking food, makes an important item in the scale of means for preserving health. This matter has been considerably anticipated and superseded while considering the subject of exercise; yet something more may be said, and the substance of previous remarks reiterated, so as to leave no chance for misapprehension or forgetfulness on this subject.

Labor is intended to mean close and intent application to business, whether of a bodily or mental character. No labor should be attempted while the nervous system is intensely engaged in the process of digestion. And as the time of this intensity is during the first hour after a meal is finished, no labor should be performed during that hour, If a laborer commence hard work immediately after eating, the action of his nervous energies is distracted; partly drawn toward the stomach, and partly forced in the direction of the muscular system. By this unnatural, forced action of the nerves, the digestive process is impaired; the food is not thoroughly broken up by, and mixed with, the gastric juice. By this unnatural operation, the food is comparatively unprepared for all the rest of the process. The chyme and chyle must be imperfectly formed, and the system, so far as each such meal is concerned, imperfectly nourished. Besides this, the forcing of the muscles to exertion against the natural inclination of the nerves to supply the necessary power, gradually impairs the power and activity of the muscular system.

The man who disregards this law will grow old faster — other things being equal — than the man who allows time for the thorough digestion of his food. It is his food which sustains him in labor; therefore, he is in duty bound to give that food the best possible opportunity to give him support. The same law prevails in dumb animals as in man. Whoever works his oxen or drives his horses immediately after their eating, will find, in the course of an experience sufficient to test the point, that his beasts, under such a management, will soon wear out; while his neighbor's beast, under a management which accords with nature's law, will be robust and endure. It is economy, then, as well as health, to yield obedience to this natural law.

Mental labor should never be attempted within one hour after a meal is finished. If a close mental application be made immediately after eating, whether at be a merchant casting accounts, or a student getting his lesson, the digestive process is impaired; the nervous energies are drawn, in a measure, away from the direction of the stomach to the brain. This unnatural action frequently causes an increased quantity of blood to be lodged on that organ, occasioning a dull, heavy headache. Sometimes it will bring on a nervous headache. The influence of this course is also very injurious to the stomach. Hundreds and thousands of students have in this way brought upon themselves dyspepsia, with its long train of untold symptoms and sufferings. Many a one has in this way broken irremediably his constitution. With too little physical exercise at the right time, and with mental labor at the wrong time, he has ruined himself for life, or brought himself to a premature grave. Many a one has gone through a regular course of education — prepared his mind for usefulness — but by having neglected the laws of his body — neglected to keep up a proper balance of action between his physical and intellectual powers- — he has rendered himself disqualified for much execution in the callings of life. His mind, though well disciplined, cannot act in this life without a body; the bodily energies are so deranged and weakened, as to hold the intellectual faculties in a state of comparative imbecility.

Students should accustom themselves to considerable daily exercise of body, in order to preserve a balance of physical and mental energy. This should be done for the sake of aiding them in making intellectual proficiency, and of preserving a good constitution for future usefulness. Their principal physical exercise should be taken on an empty stomach, i.e., just preceding a meal. Just after a meal, they should be at leisure, or amusement which requires no mental or physical exertion, for at least one hour. Then they are prepared for close study until near the time of the next meal; leaving a little space for relaxation: as also when bodily exercise precedes a meal, a few minutes' relaxation before eating should be had, that the nerves may regain their equilibrium.

But when exercise is spoken of in relation to students, that which would agitate or exhaust the body is not meant. Such exercise would be decidedly detrimental. If students would give time for eating and for digesting, they could perform a large amount of mental labor with far less time devoted to mere exercise, and that exercise of a milder character, than would otherwise be required. But every student should accustom himself to a brisk, lively, cheerful daily exercise, if he values his health. The same rule applies with equal force to every one, whatever may be his calling, whose labors are of a mental character. Under these rules, three hours of close study would be worth more than six in the ordinary way.

FOOD AND DRINKS

All our nutrition comes primarily from the vegetable kingdom. If we eat flesh, the nourishment which made that flesh came from vegetables. The nutrition from the corn on which the hog is fatted becomes assimilated into his flesh, and by eating that pork we get the nutrition of the corn, animalized, after passing through, and having been incorporated into, his system; or if we eat pork that has been fatted on dead animal matter, we get our vegetable nutrition after its having passed through two processes of assimilation. But it is proposed to speak here of taking vegetable nutrition in its original state.

This was unquestionably the original method adopted by the Creator for the nourishment of man. Man, in his original, holy state, was provided for from the vegetables of that happy garden which was given him to prune. This was the Creator's original plan; one animal was not to devour another animal for food; the eating of flesh was suffered as one of the consequences of the fall. Living on vegetable food is undoubtedly the most natural and healthy method of subsistence.

It is not intended in this small work to dwell so particularly upon the kind of food which may be most conducive to health, as upon the manner and regularity of eating. There are, however, some vegetables in common use, which ought promptly and forever to be rejected. Cucumbers, though considered a luxury, should never be eaten. They are cold, indigestible things. True, some stomachs can seem to digest them with apparent impunity: so, too, some stomachs can digest jackknives; but this does not prove that they should be used for food. The condiments with which they are usually prepared do not assist in their digestion; except by over-stimulating the stomach, which stimulating process always tends to weaken that organ. Condiments aid in digestion in the same way that alcoholic liquor aids a laborer in performing an extra task; which process always tends to weaken the system. There are other articles which might be mentioned as inappropriate for the human stomach; but a little common sense and observation will generally decide upon what is proper and what improper.

It is proper and needful that a continual sameness in diet should be avoided. It is better that there should be considerable sameness in each individual meal; but the kind of articles of which different meals are composed may with benefit be varied. The more simple the diet on the whole, the better. Complicated food, especially that which is compounded with various kinds of condiments, is bad; such as very rich puddings, cake, and pastry of various sorts. Mince pies, wedding-cake, and plum-puddings, as they are generally made, should never be introduced into the human stomach — and the prohibition need never extend beyond the human stomach, for dumb animals could not be compelled to eat them. Food should be simple, yet nutritious, and so prepared — though not with stimulating ingredients —as to be palatable — inviting to the appetite. If the food be poor or poorly prepared, the stomach will loathe it. Here is found one cause why some have not been successful in their efforts to simplify their diet; they have reduced their living to a poverty-stricken quality, by which their whole systems have become weakened. Food should be palatable and nutritious. It is not best that that kind of food should be constantly used which embraces within a given quantity the greatest amount of nutrition; but the nutritious and comparatively innutritious kinds, should be used together; for instance, sugar is too nutritious, i.e., too much nutrition in a given quantity, to be used alone as a meal; the digestive organs would soon break down with such an incumbrance. But sugar is a good article of diet when used in conjunction with articles containing less nutrition in the same quantity.

Simplicity of diet, i.e., living on simple, plain food, is exceedingly important in securing good health and a sound constitution. The great cause of the difference between the present standard of health and that of puritan times, consists in the difference in the manner of living. Then the people lived naturally; now they live artificially. Then their food was plain, homely, and simple; now it is rich, delicate, and complicated. Then the bean-porridge was the luxury; now the highly seasoned meats and the rich pastry. The children were brought up on plainer food than even their parents; now the little ones generally are invited to all the unnatural luxuries in which the parents indulge. Then a plain brown crust, even without butter, was ate with relish; now nothing but the richest dainties will meet the demand.

Fruits of various kinds are proper articles of diet in connection with other food. Apples, pears, plums, cherries, oranges, pine-apples, &c, may properly be made articles of diet, and come under the same rules and restrictions as other articles of food. They may be treated as mere luxuries to be eaten at any and all times; because they require very little effort of the digestive organs to dissolve them and extract their nutrition. It is undoubtedly better, however, that fruit should be taken as other articles of diet, at the regular time of eating, as a part of the meal. As a general rule, fruit should be taken as a part of the regular dinner. Good, ripe fruit, taken in this way, is beneficial to health by way of variety; and, if the bowels are at all sluggish, fruits are adapted to remove that difficulty.

The quantity of food which it is necessary to take at each meal is not a matter of so much importance as the regularity and simplicity of diet. Some writers on diet have undertaken to prescribe certain limits to the quantity of food to be taken, by weight. This would seem to be a difficult task. To measure out to each one a quantity suited to all the different circumstances in which he may be placed, and to all persons according to their great variety of ages and constitutions, would be a laborious undertaking indeed: and it seems to be unnecessary. Whoever will govern himself by dietetic law — eat plain food — only three times a day — give time for food to digest — take proper exercise — will find little difficulty in settling the question, how much he ought to eat. Whoever will live right, need not ask his cook to weigh out his quantum of food: only give her a chance, and Dame Nature will settle that matter, and relieve him of all such burden of mind. A person with morbid appetite may eat too much; and he should limit himself: but a perfectly healthy stomach will easily decide when it is sufficiently supplied.

Many have injured themselves by too rigidly limiting themselves in their quantity of food; so that their systems were not sufficiently nourished. In the effort to change their course of living from extreme luxury to temperance, they ran over the line, into the opposite extreme. They reduced the quantity and the quality of their food too low. By this course they reduced their health and strength, and finally perhaps concluded that their former way of living was the best. The system must have nourishment, and the quantity must be varied according to circumstances; and a perfectly healthy stomach will furnish the best index to the quantity demanded.

It is a misfortune for any one, especially for one whose health has become deranged, to keep his mind continually dwelling on the questions, what he shall eat, how much, &c, because this continued mental anxiety tends to embarrass the free action of the digestive functions, and increase the difficulty. Still he must give some attention to the subject in some way: he must hot be reckless in regard to the laws of his existence. The better way is, let him make himself intelligent on the subject of the laws of his nature, and then he can keep himself within the limits of those laws without mental effort, as well as he can keep himself within the limits of civil law when once understood.

ANIMAL FOOD

No strenuousness on this subject is intended; it is better to let each one choose for himself: yet it may not be improper that some suggestions should be made, some facts stated, and the results of experience shown, for the benefit of any who may be willing to heed. Flesh, as already intimated, composed no part of the food provided for man in his primeval state: its use came to be suffered in consequence of the fall. And if, as argued by some, the food obtained only from the vegetable kingdom is not adequate to the sustenance of man, the Creator must have made a mistake in his first arrangement for the support of his creatures. The fact that naturalists have classified man as in part a carnivorous animal, does not prove it his duty to eat flesh: because either the indications of his classification are the result of his habits of flesh-eating, or they existed before the fall, and mean nothing as relates to his mode of living. The teeth of the carnivorous animals have either conformed to their habits, or they existed in the present form before the fall, and consequently have nothing to do with their eating flesh; for it cannot be supposed that animals devoured one another in their primeval state.

One objection to eating animal food lies in the fact that it increases the proportion of our animality. When the nutrition of vegetation comes to us through the flesh of an animal, it has undergone a sort of animalization; and as it passes into our circulation the proportion of the animality in our natures is increased. A serious objection would seem to lie against such a result, for man is quite sufficiently animal without taking a course to make him more so.

The facts supporting the above statement are these. It is well known that when hunters wish to prepare their hounds for the chase, they confine the diet of those animals to flesh; and that this course does increase the savageness of their dispositions. When ancient warriors desired to give their soldiery a special fitting for the brutal battle-field, they would feed them exclusively on flesh. When the gamester at cock-fighting is preparing his fowl to win the prize, he confines him to flesh. The experiment of flesh-eating has been tried upon the cow. When she was confined to flesh food, rather than starve, she at length ate flesh; and finally lusted after it, and ate it as greedily as though she had belonged to the carnivorous race. But it changed her natural disposition to that of the tiger: she became ferocious. And she verified another general rule with meat-eaters; she lost all her teeth.

It is generally admitted among intelligent people, that eating much flesh tends to animality; and that consequently it is not well for those who devote themselves to study to indulge largely in the use of meat. This general impression is founded on sound philosophy. When we increase the proportion of our animal nature, we oppress the intellectual and moral. If students would make easy progress, they must not indulge themselves with eating much flesh; and the less the better. If any would be eminent in morals or religion, let them eat but little flesh; and the less the better. For when we increase the activity of the animal propensities, we weaken the power of the moral sentiment, and endanger the rectitude of moral action. We need to encourage and cultivate our intellectual and moral powers, rather than our carnality. We are naturally savage enough in our dispositions, and fleshly enough in out appetites, without taking a course that will increase those qualities. There can be no question but that the use of flesh tends to create a grossness of body and spirit. A reference to the history and character of different nations alone would prove this. There is certainly a grossness in the idea of one dumb animal's making food of another animal; and the idea of an intelligent being's devouring the flesh of another animate creature us grosser still. And will a person of refinement — will the advocate of moral purity and religion — will woman indulge in such luxuries?

Animal food vitiates the fluids of the system. Practical demonstration has often substantiated this statement. Take the great mass of cases which require treatment for a humor, and it will generally be found that the individuals thus affected were, themselves or their immediate predecessors, large eaters of flesh. Even the cancer can generally be traced back, either mediately or immediately, to such an origin. And what has been found to be the most effectual remedy in cases of common humor? Abstinence from eating flesh. When we feed on flesh, we not only eat the muscular fibers, but the juices or fluids of the animal; and these fluids pass into our own circulation — become our blood — our fluids, and our flesh. However pure may be the flesh of the animals we eat, their fluids tend to engender in us a humorous state of the blood. But the meat that is given us in the markets is very far from being pure. The very process taken to fit the animals for market, tends to produce a diseased state of their fluids. The process of stall feeding is a forced and unnatural process, by which the fluids become diseased; and then we eat those diseased fluids. Some of our meat is fatted in country pastures; but by the time it reaches us, the process of driving to market has produced a diseased action of the fluids.

If it be argued that these objections may lie against raw meat, but not against it when cooked, it may be answered, that if meat can be cooked so severely as to remove its juices entirely, it might be comparatively harmless; but just in proportion to those juices will be its nutrition, and also its injurious qualities; besides, if the juices could be entirely removed, who would eat the meat? and how could nourishment be obtained from it?

Animal food exposes the system more effectually to the causes of acute disease. Where the fluids are in a diseased state the ordinary causes of disease find a more easy prey. Thousands on thousands of those who have been afflicted with or have died of fevers, small- pox, cholera, &c, might probably have escaped their deadly influence if their fluids had not been vitiated by animal food. In cases of inoculation for smallpox, a dieting process is recommended, which very much mitigates the malignant character of the disease. But let an individual be inoculated who has been accustomed to simplicity and regularity of diet, and especially who has been accustomed to abstinence from animal food, and he is already dieted; he need not change his course; he is prepared to have the disease with comparative safety. The use of meat is undoubtedly a fruitful source of disease, and a means of enhancing those diseases which are unavoidable. The severest cases of worms in children may, as a general rule, be found among the greatest meat-eaters.

The vitiated state of the fluids is often seen in the character of wounds. In those whose fluids are pure, wounds heal readily. Smooth-cut wounds, if rightly treated, will heal by what is called "the first intention," or the first effort of nature: while in those whose fluids are vitiated, there is a liability to extensive inflammation and ulceration. In cases of rough wounds and bruises, where the fluids are pure, nature gets up a cure with remarkable speed; but in those whose fluids are corrupted, the process of cure is generally long protracted, and sometimes exceedingly obstinate and unmanageable. The following extract contains testimony on this point: —

"FLESH-EATING AND VEGETABLE-EATING. — To consider man anatomically, he is decidedly a vegetable-eating animal. He is constructed like no flesh-eating animal, but like all vegetable-eating animals. He has not claws like the lion, the tiger, or the cat, but his teeth are short and smooth, like those of the horse, the cow, and the fruit-eating animals; and his hand is evidently intended to pluck the fruit, not seize his fellow animals. What animals does man most resemble in every respect? The ape tribes: frugiverous animals. Doves and sheep, by being fed on animal food, (and they may be, as has been fully proved,) will come to refuse their natural food: thus has it been with man. On the contrary, even cats may be brought up to live on vegetable food, so they will not touch any sort of flesh, and be quite vigorous and sleek. Such cats will kill their natural prey just as other cats, but will refuse them as food. Man is naturally a vegetable-eating animal: how, then, could he possibly be injured by abstinence from flesh? A man, by way of experiment, was made to live entirely on animal food; after having persevered ten days, symptoms of incipient putrefaction began to manifest themselves. Dr. Lamb, of London, has lived for the last thirty years on a diet of vegetable food. He commenced when he was about fifty years

of age, so he is now about eighty, — rather more, I believe, — and is still healthy and vigorous. The writer of the Oriental Annual mentions that the Hindus, among whom he travelled, were so free from any tendency to inflammation, that he has seen compound fractures of the skull among them, yet the patient to be at his work, as if nothing ailed him, at the end of three days. How different is it with our flesh-eating, porter-swilling London brewers: a scratch is almost death to them."
— *Flowers and Fruits, by J. E. Dawson.*

The objections, then, against meat-eating are threefold: intellectual, moral, and physical. Its tendency is to check intellectual activity, to depreciate moral sentiment, and to derange the fluids of the body. It is a consequent of the fall, and is adapted to enhance its evils. It is not essential to physical energy and strength: if it is, then the Creator, as before stated, made a mistake when he originally gave to man for his nourishment simply the fruits of Eden.

Animal food is also too stimulating. Simple stimulus mixed with nutrition is what we not only do not need, but its tendency is injurious. Take two laboring men — one lives on meat, the other on vegetables — the meat-eater may at first be able to excel in the amount of labor performed in a given time, just as that man will excel who takes brandy with his meal; but in the long run, the man who depends on nutrition that is simple and unstimulating will endure longer and perform more.

The objections against eating flesh are, however, less forcible in the case of laborers than of those of intellectual and sedentary habits. While the laborer works off a measure of the evil influence exerted on his intellectual, moral, and physical systems, the sedentary man retains them.

In speaking of the objections to meat-eating, all kinds of flesh are not meant: fish may be excepted: and fowls are altogether less objectionable than the general run of quadrupeds. And the objections to meat-eating in general are not meant to be urged with the same strenuousness which is intended to be used in regard to other matters presented in this work: for while these may strictly be resolved into rules of natural law, those may perhaps with propriety come under rules of expediency. Matters of fact have been stated, deductions philosophically drawn, and practical demonstrations presented; and every candid reader — unbiassed by a flesh-loving appetite — can easily come to the conclusion for himself, whether it be better to eat or to dispense with flesh in his diet. The author of these suggestions has given the matter of abstinence from flesh-eating a trial of six years; and would by no means be induced to return to the use of animal food.

STIMULATING DRINKS

If we would enjoy health, all stimulants should be avoided as common drinks. They may be useful as medicines when nature falters and droops, and cannot rise and resuscitate herself; but, as a beverage, stimulating drinks should be strenuously avoided.

When stimulants are taken, the machinery of the system is hurried and driven too fast. And although by this means its activity and power may seem to be increased, yet a reaction must follow — a corresponding debility must ensue; then another stimulating draught is called for, to bring the system up again, and then another reaction must follow. By this course of things the real, natural vigor of the constitution becomes gradually, and oftentimes imperceptibly, impaired.

Hence, if we would preserve a healthy system, instead of provoking nature to unnatural action, we must furnish her with sufficient healthy nourishment, and let her regulate her own mode and speed of action. Give her nourishment, and she will furnish her own stimulus, which will be far preferable to any promptings which art can invent. Sustain her in her natural action, and not force her to unnatural speed, which must result in weakening her innate powers. To live naturally, is to live healthily; but to live artificially, is to tempt and foster disease.

Suppose a case for an illustration: a man undertakes riding a long journey; his beast naturally and easily travels at the rate of five miles the hour; he can do this day after day, with proper care and feeding, and come out bright at the end of the journey. But the foolish rider is not satisfied with this steady speed; ' it would be more to his gratification to travel much faster; so he goads up the poor animal to an unnatural speed, say eight miles an hour. He intends that forty miles shall be each day's travel; and by going five miles the hour, eight hours on the road would be required for its accomplishment. But by means of whip and spur, he performs the allotted distance in five hours, provided the abused beast do not give out before the day's work is finished. Now any one of common sense can at once judge of the ability of the animal to perform a long journey, and of his condition at the end of it, under such a system of driving. Every time his goading drives his beast faster than his natural speed, a reaction ensues; which continued process wears fast upon his natural strength.

Precisely in this way do those whose rule of living is their present gratification, treat their own animal systems. Instead of allowing nature to take her own speed, they goad her on to unwonted action, and consequently lessen her power to perform her functions, and her ability to endure her labor.

Why not let nature alone? Why interfere and jostle her

natural operations? Why spur on the noble steed to unnatural fastness, break down his constitution, and disable him for reaching the end of his journey? Besides all the wrong in the case, it is bad economy; what is gained temporarily, is lost, and much more with it, ultimately. Let nature alone, and she will temper her speed to the laws of health and endurance — she needs no whips and spurs — she asks no help. While she is able to do her own work, all help is hindrance. The animal that is driven beyond his five miles the hour by the whipping process, becomes so exhausted and dull, that even the five miles' speed cannot be performed without increasing the stimulus of the whip. So nature, by continued stimulus, becomes dull and lifeless in her operations, and cannot be kept up to the mark without goading her up more and more.

Alcoholic liquors of all kinds, whether strong beer, porter, ale, cider, or brandy, &c, are never to be taken; because, besides the danger of a drunkard's grave, they are all stimulants; they impart no nourishment to the system, but force its action to an unnatural degree. The idea that these liquors promote digestion is all a delusion. They give to the stomach an unnatural and forced action, which, while in health, it does not need; and the longer it is subjected to this driving process, the more will it depend on stimulants. When the stomach is excited in this way, the brain also is excited; and whoever uses alcoholic drinks as a beverage, is a drunkard; for no dividing-line can be drawn — no transition boundary can be made — between him who drinks moderately and him who drinks excessively.

Coffee is objectionable for a similar reason, it is a stimulant — a kind of narcotic stimulant bearing some resemblance to opium; and so powerful is its action, that it is considered and used as a most certain antidote to poisoning from opium. And it can readily be seen that unless it was an article of much power itself, it could never overpower such a poison. Coffee should never he placed on any other list than that of medicines; it never should be drank as a luxury or beverage. Mothers should never be so tender and affectionate toward their children as to give them such an article for their drink. Yet, if they are determined to gratify their tender ones at all hazards of their constitutions, they are of course at liberty to do so; or if any are disposed to treat themselves in the same way, there is no civil law against it; hut they break another law which must be met: a law of nature written on the constitution.

A French writer, Mons. A. Richard, says, "This liquor, taken warm, is an energetic stimulant; it has all the advantages of spirituous drinks, without any of their bad. results; that is to say, that it produces neither drunkenness nor all the accidents that accompany it." This is true to the very letter; it produces all the injurious stimulant effects of alcoholic liquor, except taking away men's senses and making them stagger and fall.

Dr. Colet thus describes the effect of coffee when taken in a large quantity, for a length of time: "To gastralgia" — acute pain in the stomach — "that it occasions, is united, after a variable space of time, a kind of shivering, a trembling in the left side of the breast, an uncomfortable stitch in front of this region, accompanied by pain in breathing, and in addition a general excitement, the characteristics of which are analogous to those of incipient intoxication." He tells us also that if this course is persevered in, spasms and convulsions are sometimes produced.

Dr. Cottereau says, "I have seen some young persons who have taken excessive doses of coffee to excite them to labor, fall into a state of stupidity, lose their appetite, and grow thin in an astonishing manner."

A. Saint-Arroman, to whom credit is due for furnishing the above extracts, says, "According to these counsels, given by men of skill, it is easy to comprehend that coffee is sometimes more injurious than the great consumption of it would seem to indicate. Thus, how many persons are there who would know the cause of a disease not understood, and would be less disordered, if they thoroughly knew the effects of this liquor, and the circumstances in which it cannot fail to be injurious."

It need only be added that, in the estimation of the writer of this little work — after having used it for several years, and since that having abstained from it for twelve or fifteen years — coffee, in all cases, and under all circumstances, is bad; that its stimulating qualities are decidedly injurious to the system, and ought never to be used except when required as an antidote to poison, or for some other medicinal purpose. And what makes it to be dreaded more than many other injurious things is, its evil working is so unseen and delusive. While it does not show itself like alcohol, yet its evil work is as certainly undermining the nervous system; and while it tempts us to believe that it strengthens and supports — because it excites — it slowly enervates. It affects the whole system, and especially the nervous system, by its effects on the stomach. But besides this, it creates a morbid action of the liver; especially where there is a tendency to bilious affections. It affects the circulation of the blood, and the quality of the blood itself, so that a great coffee-drinker can generally be known by his complexion; it gives to the skin a dead, dull, sallow appearance.

Coffee affects not only the body to its injury, but also the mind. It has been called an "intellectual drink," because it excites the mind temporarily to unwonted activity. "But, unfortunately," says the French writer last quoted, "it is not without great prejudice to mind and body that man procures such over-excitements. After them come prostration, sadness, and exhaustion of the moral and physical forces; the mind becomes enervated, the body languishes. To a rich imagination succeeds a penury of ideas; and if the consumer does not stop, genius will soon give place to stupidity.

The longevity of some coffee-drinkers has been sometimes urged as proof that coffee does no harm. But we might just as well bring forward the fact that some great alcohol-drinkers, or some great opium- eaters, have lived sometimes to old age, in proof that alcohol and opium are harmless luxuries. It is impossible to judge always of the evil effects of an article we are using by any immediate perceptible result. We must inquire what is its nature; and then draw our conclusions as to what will be its effect. The most violent poisons may be used, after a habit is established, with apparent impunity; such as tobacco, opium, and arsenic; and yet no one would dare to say these are harmless luxuries. They are not harmless; they expose their consumers to premature sickness, old age, and death. And they see not the breakers until they are dashed upon them.

Tea is another objectionable article, because of its stimulating properties. This is a direct and active stimulant. Its effects are very similar to those of alcoholic drinks, except that of drunkenness. Like alcohol, it gives, for a time, increased vivacity of spirits. Like alcohol, it increases, beyond its healthy and natural action, the whole animal and mental machinery; after which there must come a reaction — a corresponding languor and debility. The washwoman becomes exhausted, and must have her bowl of tea to recruit her energies, instead of giving nature a chance to recover herself. She depends upon art rather than nature, and each time lowers the standard of her own permanent strength. She accomplishes more in a short time, while her strength is artificial instead of natural, but is gradually, though perhaps imperceptibly, wearing herself out before her time. The nurse keeps herself awake nights by this artificial process; and each time, by imperceptible steps, lessens her natural strength. She thinks with the wash-woman, that tea does her good — strengthens her, because, like the rum-drinker, she feels better under its immediate effects.

The time was when ministers, instead of being largely inspired with the Holy Ghost, wrote and delivered their sermons under the inspiration of ardent spirits; but now, seeing that to be morally and physically wrong, they not infrequently labor under that artificial inspiration, which is quite as effectual, contained in tea. By this process, they gradually impair their own natural energy of body and mind.

See a party of Indies met to spend an afternoon, in a sewing-circle, it may be; toward the close of the afternoon, their fund of conversationals becomes somewhat exhausted; but soon come the tea and eatables; and notwithstanding the opposing influences of a full stomach, the drooping mind becomes greatly animated, the tongue is let loose, and the words come flowing forth like the falling drops of a great shower in summer-time. What does all this mean? Whence the cause of such a change? It is the inspiration of the strong cups of tea. Then is the time for small thoughts and many words; or it may be the sending forth of fire- brands of gossip and slander; or if, perchance, religion be the topic, the inspiring power of tea will create an excited feeling very closely resembling that produced when alcohol runs over in the form of penitential tears.

Tea, in large doses, produces convulsive motions, and a kind of intoxication. It enters into the circulation, and affects the complexion; it is not difficult to detect a great tea-drinker by looking at his skin; which loses its bright and lively cast, and puts on a deadly, lifeless, dried, and sometimes sallow appearance. It is said that in China the great tea-drinkers are thin and weak, their complexion leaden, their teeth black, and themselves affected with diabetes. Cases have not infrequently come under the immediate inspection of the writer, where tea had for years almost literally been the food and drink; especially of seamstresses, who would sit up late nights. In such cases, about the only remedy would be, to prohibit the further use of it. But generally this prohibition would be no longer heeded than while being uttered; for their dependence on it, and love for it, could not be easily broken up; and but small compensation in some cases would seem to be gained by its discontinuance; for tea had almost eaten them up; leaving little more than bone and sinew, and a few scraps of dried flesh.

In short, whoever uses tea or coffee as a common drink, spends his money for that which does him not only no good, but evil, and that continually. They are both innutritious, and stimulating to a degree which it is difficult for their devotees to calculate. Now which shall we do? Abstain, and bring under this evil appetite, or will we gratify it? Will we deny ourselves, and derive the incalculable benefit as a compensation, or recklessly go on, and take the consequences? Will young ladies and gentlemen treat their physical and mental systems lawfully, and save to themselves a good constitution, or will they, at all hazards, indulge themselves in unlawful appetites, and have no principle by which to govern themselves, but their own gratification? Will they have regard to their own benefit, and that of coming generations, or will they, like the devotee to the intoxicating bowl, live for to-day, and let to-morrow provide for itself?

NOURISHING DRINKS

As it has been said before, so let it be repeated — which should be, at all times in health, a standing rule — -give to nature a sufficient nutrition, and she will furnish her own stimulus, far better than anything which art can do. Support nature, and let art go begging. Live naturally, and not artificially. The natural inquiry will now be, what shall we drink?

Cocoa is a healthy drink. That which comes in pound and half-pound papers makes a very good drink; but on account of its oily nature, which is objectionable, the cracked nut of cocoa is preferable; but caution is necessary not to make it too strong, because it contains a large amount of nutrition in a small compass, and may oppress the stomach and produce headache. The cracked nuts and shells, which come in bags of about thirty pounds, make the most convenient form for use. This mixture, made in moderate strength, say, according to the following proportion and rule, is a nutritious, healthy drink. Take half common tea-cupful of this cocoa-mixture, and add one quart of cold water; boil moderately for about six hours, adding more water to supply the portion which boils away; it is fit then for use by adding milk, or cream, and sugar. This makes a good substitute for coffee in the morning, and the same or simple shells in place of tea in the evening. There are various nourishing, healthy drinks, of a domestic character, such as bread-coffee, and others, which it is not important to describe or recommend.

Hot drinks of any kind are objectionable. They excite by the force of heat, and then debilitate the stomach. They should only be taken about blood- warmth. Some persons accustom themselves to drink hot milk and water; this is objectionable on account of its heat. Moderately warm water, of itself, without considerable milk or cream, if taken to much extent, is also weakening to the stomach. Warm drinks generally expose one to colds.

Large quantities of any kind of drinks should be avoided. Even cold water maybe taken too largely. Much depends upon habit; if we allow ourselves in the custom of drinking much, we shall want much; if we accustom ourselves to drink but little, we shall want but little. The objection to a large quantity is this: it distends the stomach beyond its natural dimensions, and therefore weakens it; it also dilutes the gastric juice, and therefore weakens that. One or two common tea-cups of any kind of drink, taken with our meals, is sufficient. If we take more, it weakens the gastric juice, and injures the digestive process. Laborers, at their meals, and between meals, are inclined to drink far too much. Their thirst on the whole is no less for drinking so largely, and they weaken themselves by it. Besides, in hot weather, many are seriously injured, and even destroyed sometimes, by too large quantities of cold water. If they want to drink often, they must confine themselves to very small quantities at a time.

Unfermented beers — root, hop, and ginger beers — are healthy drinks, if not taken too largely. Soda

drinks, in the form of soda powders, or from soda fountains, are also healthy. The carbonic acid gas which they impart to the stomach does not excite, but is a moderate tonic.

PARTICULAR DIRECTIONS

Parents have a responsibility in regard to their offspring originating prior to their birth. Their own state of health — the health of father and mother- — has a very important bearing upon the constitutions of their yet unborn children. If a father's nervous system has been marred and broken by habits which are at war with nature's law, the generations following him will be more or less unhappily affected. While, then, he is doing wrong to himself, he is doing wrong, and bringing suffering upon his posterity. If a mother's system has been weakened by violations of law, her children, prior to birth, will be obliged to participate with her in suffering the penalty. And having received the inheritance of disease or debility before birth, they must, more or less, be the partakers of it through life. Parents have also a heavy responsibility on them, touching the moral character given to their children before birth. If parents are accustomed to undue indulgence in any of the natural propensities — in eating or drinking, or any other animal appetite — their children are sure, prior to birth, to inherit appetites of the same kind, possessing a similar degree of undue activity.

In the same way, previously to birth, children are affected in their dispositions. A child, after birth, and more or less through life, will give a living illustration of the feelings and immediate character of his mother during the period of her pregnancy. If the mother, during that period, especially the latter part of it, indulges a gloomy, evil-foreboding state of mind, her child will give proof of it in after life. If she indulge a peevish, or fretful, or crying disposition, her child will give her ample testimony to the fact after birth. Some have inherited directly from a mother an almost unconquerable appetite for strong drink; others, an almost uncontrollable inclination to theft; not because their mothers, in all cases, were habitual drinkers or thieves, but because they suffered those feelings to affect them strongly sometime during their pregnancy. Many physicians would deny the truth of these statements; but no one who has taken the pains of observing facts touching this matter will be found in that category; for facts are unconquerable things. The inspired proverb, "Train up a child in the way he should go, and when he is old he will not depart from it," contains a great practical truth as a general rule: but under the most judicious discipline, the child will bear, in greater or less degree, the moral complexion which his mother gave him before she gave him birth.

Fathers, as well as mothers, and all those with whom a mother may associate, are involved in this responsibility. The father should remember that his manner and treatment of his wife during her pregnancy has much to do with the disposition she may possess during that period. He should be careful to remove, so far as possible, every source, real or imaginary, of uneasiness, unhappiness, peevishness, or gloominess, from her way. He should take pains to make her happy and cheerful; and see that every appetite which conies up is, if possible, forthwith gratified. If that appetite should be for strong drink, it had better be gratified to the full, rather than (hat she give, by that continued longing, an indelible imprint of that kind upon her offspring. In the light of these truths, what tremendous responsibilities are evidently laid upon parents. But as this work relates mainly to physical health, further remarks on that of morals might seem irrelevant.

The object of these remarks is to elevate the standard of general health in the rising generation. One great cause of the feebleness of constitution with which the great body of community is at the present day afflicted, may be found in the total ignorance or recklessness of parents and guardians of the laws of health as applied to those under their care. To look in upon many domestic circles, and see how the children are managed, is enough to move a heart of marble, with sorrow for the children, and with indignation towards their parents. The children may be seen, about every hour in the day, with a lunch of bread, or pie, or cake, in hand. Their young and tender stomachs are kept in continual confusion and toil.

Children should eat only three times a day. They should be brought under the same dietetic rules which are laid down for all persons. It requires about as much time for their organs to digest food as is required for grown persons. And if the digestive process be hurried and confused, their food docs not nourish them as well, and they cannot grow as strong and robust. Little new- born infants' constitutions are not infrequently ruined for life, by mismanagement. Because the child cries a little, it must be dosed with a little peppermint, or anise-essence, or paregoric, or some other stimulating article, which begins at once to derange his stomach; and through his stomach, his whole system is injured, and probably for life. And if the inquiry should be made, in after years, what can be the cause of such a feeble, slender constitution? an enlightened observer would be able to reveal the secret, by showing the treatment received in infancy.

A systematic diet should always he adopted by mothers and nurses at the very dawn of the child's existence. In the first place, after birth, a little cold water only should be put into the child's mouth. The habit of beginning to give some stimulant, as though the Creator of the child had given it only half life enough, is perfectly murderous: instead of giving it a chance to live of itself, a course is taken which is adapted to kill it; or if not kill it, to maim its little constitution for life. If the writer of this could be heard, he would "cry aloud, and spare not," in the ear of every nurse, with the little being in her arms, LET THAT CHILD LIVE! If it be necessary to give the child any nourishment before it can obtain it from the mother, it might take a little slippery elm water, or something of that mild and simple nature: but if it can draw its first nourishment from the fountain which the Author of its being has provided, it is better.

Babes should be nursed but three times a day. This may seem a preposterous rule; but let us reason together upon it. The food which Nature has provided for the child is adapted to its age and capacity for digesting; and it requires about the same length of time for the infant to digest its meal as it does the man of ripe age to digest his; and the various steps in the digestive process are the same in both cases. Then if five hours are required to complete the process well, why disturb it till it is finished? By letting the child have only its regular breakfast, dinner, and supper, it digests its food well, and is well nourished by it. But adopt the course usually taken, and the little one's stomach is kept confused and oppressed, and its system is but half nourished from the same quantity of food which would be requisite under a regular system. As infants are usually treated, they are subject to repeated vomiting, colic, and, not infrequently, fits; and the cause is obvious: the stomach has been overloaded. Only feed infants right, and there is no reason why they should vomit any more than grown persons. What danger can there be of a child's suffering from want of food before the expiration of the five hours between meals, when they not infrequently go from twelve to twenty-four hours, and sometimes longer, after birth, before they take any substantial nourishment? The idea that a child will suffer hunger, if it do not take food oftener than once in five hours during the day, is all nonsense; and worse than this, great injury is done by such a notion. The "little and often" system is destructive — contrary to the laws of health — contrary to true philosophy and reason; and should forever be abandoned.

If infants from the first were treated in this way, they would not only be more healthy, but altogether more quiet, and easy to be taken care of. Then, instead of putting the child to the breast to stop its mouth and get rid of its crying, it would feel better, and be far less likely to cry. And generally, instead of worrisome nights — usually caused by a disturbed stomach — it would sleep quietly till morning; and the mother with it. The food of the infant, taken just before it sleeps, or in the night, interferes with its quiet sleep; just as that of any other individual, from a similar cause, is disturbed. This experiment has been tried, and proved successful: let others try it.

When children are old enough to take solid food, they should have only three meals a day. If they eat oftener, their stomachs will be deranged, and their food will not so well nourish them. If any mother will take pains to look at the laws of digestion, she will at once see that no child can take food oftener than once in five hours without interfering with a previous meal, and injuring the healthful operation of the digestive organs. Those children who have been brought up on the exclusive system of eating but three times a day, have been proved to be more than ordinarily strong and healthy. While other children have been afflicted with worms, colic, choleramorbus, and a host of other ailments common to children generally, they have escaped.

Why, then, will mothers suffer their children to. violate the laws of their natures, and expose themselves to suffer the penalty of those violated laws? Will a mother have such a tender concern for her offspring's gratification, as to suffer it to destroy its own comfort and health, and perhaps life? It is often said, "My child has no appetite for breakfast; therefore it must have a lunch before dinner." But this is a sure way of prolonging the difficulty: the child will never be likely to have an appetite for breakfast, as long as this irregular and unlawful course is indulged; and especially as long as the child knows that he may depend on the precious lunch. Let the child go from breakfast time till dinner time, and it will not be long before he will eat his regular breakfast. If parents would secure for their children a healthy appetite and a sound constitution, let them rigidly insist on their eating but three times a day, using simple food, and having other things in keeping with nature's laws; and, so far as all human means are concerned, they may be sure of accomplishing their purpose.

The almost continual hankering for food which many children seem to have, arises wholly from a habit of constant eating. If their eating were reduced to a regular habit, their appetite would become regular. But this irregular appetite is not natural; it is created, and unhealthy. If we get into a habit of eating seven times a day, we shall hanker after food as many times. If we once establish a habit of eating but three times a day, we shall want food only as many times. Now, what will mothers and nurses do? Will they begin with the infant by a regular system, and continue it? or will they go on in the old beaten path, to the injury of those they profess to love and cherish? Will they make a mock of parental love and fondness, by unrestrained and unlimited indulgence? or will they love so sincerely as to keep the child from every hurtful thing? That pretended love, which, knowing the evil consequences, at all hazards, seeks only to gratify, proves its own falseness. Shame — SHAME on that mother's love which passes heedlessly by her child's chief and ultimate good, to indulge it in a momentary gratification, or to save herself the trouble of controlling its solicitations! Shame on that mother's humanity even, whose refined and tender sympathy cannot refuse indulgence where health, and, it may be, life, are at stake! If mothers and fathers have a substantial affection for their offspring, let them manifest it under the dictates of reason and common sense — let them seek their permanent good. If those having the care of children would be able to give a final account of their guardianship in peace, let them, next to their morals, seek for those under their charge, soundness of constitution. And in doing this, they do perhaps as much for their morals as could be done through any other means; for physical and moral health are closely allied.

TO LITERARY INSTITUTIONS

There is no class of persons who are under higher obligations to observe the laws of health, than those who are connected, whether as teachers or pupils, with literary institutions. Thousands have been ruined for life, so far as the enjoyment of health is concerned, and lost to the world, with all their native talents and acquired abilities, by violating those laws. Whereas, by attention and obedience to them, a balance between the healthy action of body and mind might have been preserved, and themselves and the world would have enjoyed the avails of their existence. Young men and young ladies enter upon a course of education with good health, and long before that course is finished their constitutions give way, and they are obliged to retire from study: or, if able to finish their education, they have scarcely physical energy enough left to apply their mental resources to any practical purpose. To effect a change which shall obviate this evil, will require the attention both of teachers and students.

Students should live on simple food; and remember to "eat to live, and not live to eat." To gormandize is beneath the dignity of one who has mind enough to make it worth while to submit it to a process of culture: indeed, a man who has the soul of an intellectual being will never do it. Students should avoid those things which are hard to digest. They should have food that is palatable, and well, yet with simplicity, prepared.

The less animal food — even none at all — the better. They should rigidly and scrupulously confine themselves to three — if not to two — meals a day; and for reasons given explicitly under Dietetic Rules. They should never apply their minds to study or reading at least for one hour after their meal is finished: but they should make themselves amused and cheerful in some way which neither requires the effort of body or mind: they should be at leisure, and endeavor to enjoy themselves. The reason for this course, as before stated, is, that if the nervous energies, required in the digestive process, are called away to some physical or intellectual effort, great injury is done to the digestive department. From this cause, and perhaps mainly this, thousands on thousands have either entirely broken down, or rendered themselves sufferers for life.

After one hour from the time 'the meal is finished, they may with safety set themselves down to study; i.e., if they have eaten with such moderation as all students ought to use: if not, they should wait longer; — yes, if they will not eat properly, let them retire from the institution, which is no place for gluttons, and devote themselves to corporeal labor — labor at the anvil, or in the western wilds, felling trees, where they could practice engorgement with comparative impunity. After spending about half an hour in thoroughly masticating their meal — being careful not to spend that time in too much talking, which not only interferes with mastication, but may agitate the mind, as would be the case in all argumentative conversation — and then one hour in gentle amusement or cheerful leisure, they are ready to bind their whole mental force to study. Under this arrangement, six hours a day of study will accomplish more in the long run than twelve hours in the ordinary way.

Exercise is another duty of students. It is exceedingly important that a balance between the mental and physical energies should be maintained; otherwise the body withers under its superincumbent weight. To preserve this balance while the mind is advancing, and the body untasked, artificial exercise must be instituted; for bodily strength cannot be promoted without some kind of bodily exertion.

The best time for exercise for students is about an hour before meal times; so as to give about three- fourths of an hour for hard labor, and a quarter of an hour to rest, before eating. Exercise in this way can be taken once, twice, or three times a day, as circumstances may require. The length of time devoted to exercise, and the severity of the effort which each one requires, cannot be defined by certain rules: the constitution and circumstances of each individual, aided by common sense, must determine. But every individual student requires some exercise; and it should be taken sufficiently prior to a following meal to give a little respite from exertion just previous to sitting down to eat. A division of time, between each meal, something like the following, may do as a general rule: spend half an hour in eating, one hour in leisure, two and a half hours in close study, and one hour in labor; leaving off in season to get the system calm before the next meal.

The kind of exercise to be taken may properly be a matter of inquiry. To settle upon any one kind for universal application, may be difficult. A mechanic's shop exercise may be very beneficial for body and mind. At any rate, it should be something which is adapted to give not only exercise to the muscular system, but, if possible, at the same time, a. source of amusement. Making trunks and boxes may secure this object. Sawing or chopping wood, however profitable it may be, may require too severe exertion, and may not prove to be very much amusement to the mind. The bowling alley, aside from the odium of its general character, its bewitching charms, and its tendencies to various kinds of dissipation, might afford a most desirable method of promoting muscular strength and mental exhilaration. Exercise in the line of agricultural pursuits, when it can be had, is, perhaps, everything considered, the best kind. In the use of this, there is the advantage of the open air, the smell of vegetation, the effluvia from the ground, and the vigorous action of the muscles of the arms and chest. This last benefit — one which may be had in other modes of exercise also — is very important generally, and especially where there is any tendency to falling in of the chest and Jung affection.

Walking is another kind of exercise generally employed; but it is one of very little service generally: it is better than nothing, but very insufficient. It only calls into exertion the lower limbs, which least need exercise, while the muscles of the chest and abdomen, which need them most, are not called into exertion. Horseback exercise has the same deficiency. At female schools some method should be chosen for exercise which combines the three important considerations above mentioned, namely, general muscular exertion, adapted to their strength, mental exhilaration, and the special action of the arms and trunk. Jumping the rope is too exciting and severe. A bowling alley for young ladies, who of course would never allow themselves to become dissipated, would be an excellent exercise and amusement for them. Let all students remember that if they would preserve good health, THEY MUST EXERCISE; and that in doing this, they also give vigor and vivacity to the intellect, as well as energy and health to the body.

The managers of literary institutions have a great responsibility in this matter. If they would secure the physical and intellectual welfare of those under their care, which doubtless they would, they must put themselves to the trouble of providing for and regulating means to accomplish that object.

Provision should be made for the exercise of their students. Means for agricultural exercise should be provided, if possible, for that portion of the year in which it is practicable. A mechanic's shop, or something to subserve the same purpose, should be provided for the winter season; and a requirement on every student to attend on this important duty, should be established; so that no loafer should find an easy passport through any literary institution.

Recitations should be so arranged as to accommodate the periods allotted to eating and digesting food, and those allotted to labor and relaxation. A recitation should never be required just preceding or just succeeding a meal. If it immediately precede a meal, the nervous energies have been drawn so intently to the mental effort, that they cannot at once be diverted and drawn toward the digestive effort. Therefore, a short space should be granted for relaxation from any active employment of the nervous system, immediately preceding a meal. If the recitation immediately succeed a meal, the process of digestion is interrupted. It would be far better that recitations should be so arranged as to come somewhere within the period allotted to close study. Then there would be no interference with the natural action of the system. But to go into a recitation-room just after a meal, is a violation of law, which is perfectly suicidal; and to be forced there by academic law, is gradual manslaughter.

And now the important question is, will the managers of literary institutions regulate this matter so as not to stand in the way of their students' obeying the laws of their being? Will they hinder, or will they facilitate, their employing the proper method of securing health of body and mind? Will they aid in keeping up such a balance between mental and physical power, that there may be a prospect that the world will be benefited by the existence of their institutions?

The food and drinks also, which are furnished, should be adapted to the best interests of their students. If meats be set aside, pains should be taken to furnish a palatable and wholesome vegetable diet. And as coffee and tea should never see the inside of any apartment of a literary institution, nourishing drinks should be furnished in their place. Every institution's guardians should most earnestly recommend, if not require, ten o'clock to be the hour for closing study and for retiring to rest; for there is nothing gained, but much lost, by studying after that hour of night. It is generally admitted by medical men, that sleep is worth more before than after midnight; that two hours' good sleep before twelve o'clock is worth more than four after that hour.

TO PROFESSIONAL MEN

Those who accustom themselves to intellectual labor require habits of living somewhat different from those who are engaged in pursuits of a physical character. Though all should strictly obey the laws of their natures, physical and intellectual, yet, while some habits of living may be lawful, they may not be, under certain conditions in life, expedient; and indeed what may be lawful for one, under certain circumstances, may not be lawful for another under other circumstances. For instance, as before stated, a person engaged in farming can bear the evil effects of animal food better than one of sedentary and literary habits. Since meat-eating, according to general admission tends to oppress and check mental development, it becomes inexpedient, if not unlawful, for persons devoted strictly to intellectual pursuits, to practice it. It is doubtless inexpedient for any to use it; but in the case of those whose skill and usefulness depend upon an unclouded and active intellect, this inexpediency comes near the range of moral obliquity.

For a sample of the effects of meat-eating, on a large scale, upon the intellect, see the difference between the French and English, in regard to their habits and character.

The English are inclined to gluttony; they are enormous meat-eaters; they take meat largely at each of their meals. They are generally inclined to be of the lymphatic temperament; a consequence of habitual stuffing with roast-beef, beef-steaks, and plum- puddings. And what is the effect upon the mass of mind? While we find some highly gifted, commanding, and high-toned geniuses, the mass are stupid and comparatively unintelligent.

The French live principally on vegetables; they generally possess the nervous temperament; a temperament adapted to literary and intellectual habits. They have quick and energetic minds. They have a large flow of spirits, great vivacity and cheerfulness, and are remarkably effective and productive in their mental character. It is well known that a very large proportion of various scientific works have originated from France. The science of medicine, with various collateral sciences, is highly indebted to the wakeful genius and indefatigable zeal of French intellect for its advancement.

Professional and literary men should live on simple, nutritious, and regular diet. The less exciting their food, the better; the less meat — if none at all — the better; in short, they should observe all the rules of diet previously laid down. They should by no means use stimulating drinks. Their nervous systems are more severely taxed than many other classes of men: hence the absolute necessity of economizing the nervous strength; and if they would preserve that, they must not suffer their nerves to be artificially and unnaturally excited. They should have wholesome nourishment, and then let nature herself supply her own well- balanced excitement.

The clergymen of this country, in days long since — as now in England — were accustomed to prepare and preach their sermons under, and in demonstration of, ardent spirit. Now, among us, this method is abandoned; but there is a substitute which answers precisely the same purpose, and is even better; for when the ardent was used too freely — which not infrequently occurred — the subject would reel under the weight of his accumulated ideas; while the substitute equally inspires the brain, without causing the zigzag and horizontal motions. That substitute is tea: or, it may be, coffee. The nature and effects of these articles have been already examined, and it is not necessary to dwell upon them here.

When the writer was a settled pastor, a few years since, in a neighboring town, he was accustomed to have, on entering his study, extreme nervous depression — sinking of the nervous energies — insomuch that it was impossible to make any mental effort while in that state; a bowl of tea, therefore — in accordance with previous habits — would be ordered; on taking which, the extreme depression would immediately pass away, and a most cheerful and happy flow of spirits would take its place. Under this a sermon could easily be prepared; 'and on the Sabbath, under the same kind of stimulus, it could be preached. But a little time of such violation of law developed the fearful fact that nervous debility and depression were rapidly increasing — that the more stimulus that was taken, the more must be taken to meet the demand. Hence, the tea was abandoned entirely; and very soon the complaint disappeared, and has returned no more. This is an illustration only of facts which always will exist in every instance of tea-drinking under similar circumstances, whether they be readily perceived or not. How much better in every case, and especially in that of ministers, that they depend, in all their intellectual labors, on the real, substantial, and uniform inspiration of nature, than upon the spurious, fitful, debilitating excitement of some foreign stimulant. How much better that the ministers of Christ, under such solemn and awful responsibilities as the preaching of the gospel involves, lean on the divine energy of the Holy Ghost, than on the transient energy of some artificial excitement; nay, how profane and wicked is such a departure from nature and from nature's God.

The injurious effects of tea and coffee cannot be resisted by the habits of professional men, as much as by the habits of the laboring classes. They must either abandon them altogether, or bow down as slaves to

appetite, and take the consequences. They must abandon them, or consent to have less health of body and mind, and die sooner. See the sallow complexion and trembling hand of the barrister, especially as he advances in life, who, instead of living naturally, has lived artificially all his days; will he continue to barter his highest earthly good for such pottage? He may live to old age; and so may the drunkard.

TO LABORING MEN

Remarks under the head, "Time for Labor," supersede the necessity of extended remarks under the present one. If laboring men would endure long and accomplish much, they must work and live, temperately.

Some men work too hard; and by this means violate a law of their physical nature. This is poor economy. Though for a day a man accomplish more, yet in the end, he is certainly a loser. But temperate labor is both healthy and curative in its effects on the animal system. If the hosts of dyspeptics and consumptives could turn farmers, they might dispense with drugs and doctors, and recover their health. But even farmers themselves may utterly destroy their health and constitutions by excessive and ill-managed labor. To subject one's self to a severity of labor which the strength and constitution cannot endure, is a violation of physical law, which, sooner or later, will bring in its train a penalty apportioned to the amount of transgression.

Another way in which labor may be made injurious, is by inattention to the laws of digestion. Take the case of the farmer for an illustration. Though the amount of daily labor performed by him is not sufficient of itself to injure him, yet by ignorance or disregard of the nature of the digestive process, he may do himself great injury. One way of injuring himself may be rapid eating; so that his food is no more than half masticated and half mixed with saliva. That food can comparatively do him but very little good. Or if he take sufficient time to eat, and then immediately set himself about hard labor, the process of digestion in the stomach becomes deranged and imperfect. Hence, his system is not nourished and sustained; or else he is obliged to overload his stomach with food in order to get sufficient support. But let him take ample time for eating, and. then spend one hour in digesting before he shall put himself down to hard labor, and he will soon find himself a gainer in health, and in the amount of labor ultimately performed. Take the farmer, with his dozen hands, in haying-time, it may be; they hurry down a heavy dinner, then go out immediately to mowing grass or pitching hay; while all their nervous energies are needed in the digestive process, they are forcing them away from their duty to the muscular system. The men and their work move heavily; and at the close of day they feel exhausted and overdone. But let this same farmer with his men change his course; they eat deliberately, they spend one hour in doing some light matter, and then apply themselves closely to work until the next meal. In this way they give time to masticate, time for the stomach to act, and then they work with ease, and despatch their work with much greater energy and speed; and at the close of the day they find themselves much less exhausted. Every man who knows how to manage beasts of burden, and studies economy, takes the same course with them which is here recommended for laboring men. When men or horses live and labor in this way, they ordinarily eat less, are in better condition, do more work, and endure longer.

Laboring men should also eat temperately. They are under no necessity for using animal food. They can be amply nourished on vegetable diet; else the provision made for Adam and Eve before the fall was a failure. But whatever they eat should be simple, nourishing, and palatable. They should eat moderately, and not overload their stomachs. If they eat too largely, the stomach is oppressed, and requires a longer time to perform its functions. Some are in the habit of taking luncheons between meals. They often say they want a full stomach to lean over; this is bad philosophy, for reasons which need not here be repeated. If they lunch habitually, of course when luncheon-time comes, they feel a faintness at the stomach. And so it would be if they were to eat ten times a day; and if they habituate themselves to only three meals a day, they will suffer no more, nor even so much. Three meals a day is as much as they can lawfully dispose of; and when they take more, they are obliged to violate an important law of the animal economy. They should be careful that they do not allow their supper to come near bedtime; supper should come in season for digestion. Then on rising in the morning, the head and body feel clear and active. Let laboring men adopt these suggestions, and they will find them much to their interest and happiness.

GENERAL DIRECTIONS

Sleep is as important to body and mind as food is for the general system. Without it, the health of the most robust would fail, and even life itself in time wither away. Some need more sleep than others, perhaps, under the same circumstances. But those who are destined to labor in body or in mind, need more sleep than those who 'are not exposed to fatigue. And those who are engaged in bodily labor, generally require more than those who devote themselves to that which is intellectual.

Laboring men should give themselves ample time for sleep. They should retire to rest about nine or ten o'clock at night. Nine, perhaps, is the best hour, but never in any ordinary case, should they sit up later than ten. They need, as a general rule, seven or eight hours of sleep. And sleep before midnight is generally considered worth more than sleep for the same length of time after midnight. They should rise in the morning about four or five o'clock.

Professional, literary, and mercantile men should give themselves time to rest the mind. They ought never to allow themselves to be awake after ten o'clock at night. Many may suppose that by laboring over their books or other business till eleven or twelve o'clock, they gain time and money; but this is a grand mistake. When men undertake to cheat themselves, they always get a bad bargain. Dame Nature is jealous of her rights; and whoever will be so unwise as to trample them under their feet, will, sooner or later, be made to pay damages.

If we want health and ability to endure, we must obey law by giving sufficient time, and the right time, for sleep. If any would shorten his time of sleep, let him not put off the hour of retirement, but rise earlier than the ordinary hour in the morning.

Sleep, to be quiet and refreshing, should be on an empty stomach; that is, the first steps in the process of digestion should be accomplished before retirement. Supper should be the lightest meal of the day, and should be taken at least two hours before bed-time. Some are in the habit of eating fruit after supper, and frequently late in the evening. Strong stomachs may dispose of fruit under such circumstances without apparent injury, but weak ones will suffer more or less from such a course. The better way is not to take anything, even the mildest fruit, after supper. The stomach should be allowed the privilege of rest, as well as the rest of the body. Dreams are generally the result of luncheons and suppers late in the evening. The revelations of night visions are doubtless, in many instances, the result of late suppers, producing involuntary somnambulism.

Another rule, indispensable to good health, is, never to sleep on feather-beds. One objection to them is, they are non-conductors of the various gases which are thrown off from the body, and are also gathered around it from the atmosphere. The tendencies of some of these gases are adapted, among other evils, to generate fevers. Owing to the non-conducting quality of these beds, these gases are accumulated, and are very detrimental to the system. Another objection to them is, they are the general reservoir of the various exhalations of the different bodies which have been lodged on them. They possess the power of retaining all the effluvia and humors which may have been gathered from those who have occupied them. Hence, feather- beds should be rejected, and husk, palm-leaf, or hair mattresses, should be adopted in their place.

ON BATHING

Cleanliness is a very important means of health. Some persons in low life, and some foreigners, are practically great lovers of dirt; and at the same time they have good health and sound constitutions: but they are none the better for their filthiness. Their good health may be the result alone of their plain living; while those in higher life,' with all their cleanliness and ventilation, destroy themselves with their luxuries. But when the cholera and other violent epidemics appear, their most fearful footsteps are traced in those districts and families where filth abounds. Every person ought to be accustomed to periodical bathing, or at least to occasional bathing. The pores of the skin are likely to become choked and impervious without it. Without occasional bathing the surface of the body becomes covered with a dirty and offensive substance, which prevents the action of the cutaneous vessels. Washing the surface from such accumulations is very important both for the flavor and the health of the body: for when the skin is thus coated, the whole system is affected by it: the natural exhalations which are adapted to purify the blood and fluids generally, are thrown back upon the system; and some or all of the internal organs become oppressed. Persons having an obstructed skin are more liable to fevers and pestilential diseases. An obstructed skin is frequently produced by a sudden cold; by which the internal system becomes oppressed, and a fever ensues, unless the obstruction be speedily removed. A bath to meet such an emergency is necessary. A warm bath perhaps when the action of the system is feeble, possessing but little power of reaction; but where the system is more vigorous, promising to react so as to bring up a glow of warmth and a gentle perspiration, a cold bath may be the best.

The kind of bath to be used is of some consequence. Sea water may be the best for those in general who have been unaccustomed to the atmosphere of the sea shore. It may be the best for any whose surface is too cold, lax, and flaccid, throwing off perspiration too profusely, or that which is clammy and morbid. Sea-bathing, cold or warm, as the individual may be able to bear it, accompanied with dry friction, in such cases, may prove very beneficial, A fresh water bath is unquestionably best where a fever, or a tendency to a fever, exists.

A cold or warm bath should be selected in accordance with circumstances and facts relating to the state of general constitution, present strength, or the nature of an existing morbid affection. As before remarked, as a general rule, a warm bath may be the better one when the general strength is too feeble to admit of a reaction of the system under the influence of cold water; while a cold one may be better where a tolerably vigorous habit exists. A cold bath may also be preferable, as a general thing, when resorted to as a luxury, or for the purpose of preserving health. The cold itself is a tonic to the skin, and through the skin, to the entire system: while the general tendency of warm water upon the surface is weakening. When a limb is inflamed, we bathe it freely in warm water to reduce its action; i.e., to weaken the present excited action of its vessels.

The frequency of bathing is a matter of some interest. This depends much upon the constitution, health, habits, and employment of each individual. Those who live on meats and oily substances have much more occasion for frequent baths than those of different habits. If persons would so regulate their habits of living as to keep the fluids of their systems pure, they would have much less occasion for frequent bathing. Hence no specific rule can be given for bathing, either as a preservative, restorative, or a luxury; common sense and circumstances must determine its frequency.

Too frequent bathing, however, is decidedly injurious. Although hundreds perhaps suffer for want of bathing, while one is injured by its frequency, yet there is such a thing as making too free use of a good thing. A person may bathe so often as to materially weaken himself in the course of time. Any one must be very filthy to need a bath every day. And if a bath be used every day by one who only needs one once or twice a week, and this course is persisted in for a great length of time, much damage to the system must accrue. Very many, doubtless, have been greatly injured in this way, though that injury may not have been attributed to such a cause.

Too frequent bathing does injury by stimulating the pores of the skin too much. When the skin acts naturally, it constantly throws off, by insensible perspiration or exhalation, a substance which it is necessary the system should part with for the continuance of life and health. When, from any cause, that exhalation is impeded, the system suffers by being oppressed with that which should be thrown off. But if the skin be made too active, it throws off too much — more than is required, and more than the system can afford to spare: hence the system is gradually weakened. And though years may pass before this undue waste be perceived, yet it will sooner or later discover itself. Not infrequently has the writer been called to prescribe for debilitated, rickety children, when little else could or needed to he done except to proscribe the use of too frequent baths and washings. Some mothers are so excessively afraid of their little ones being dirty, they will bathe and wash them several times a day. Such a course is liable to be very disastrous, especially when warm water is used. When children are washed for cleanliness, cold water should be used; but even that should not be applied to the whole body so often as every day, if the strength and health of the child be an object.

A letter has been recently received from the much honored ex-president, John Quincy Adams, answering some inquiries in relation to his experience on bathing, in which he says he has practiced it in a variety of forms and ways, "from first to second childhood" — an "experience during more than three score years and ten." He says, "I continued it until within the last four or five years, when I found it no longer agreeing with my health, but operating rather unfavorably to it. Medical friends, and particularly my very ancient friend, the late Dr. Waterhouse, advised me to disuse it; and my experience confirming his admonitions, I have, with great reluctance, entirely renounced it." He adds, "and I parted from it as from a dear and deeply regretted friend. Though no longer able to enjoy it myself, I can very cheerfully recommend it, not only the practice of bathing, but of swimming, to all my friends under the age when King David could get no heat."

There can be little doubt but that the fascinating luxury of bathing has sometimes led to such an undue use of it, as gradually to waste the physical energies, and induce premature old age. While the system possesses the vigor of youth and manhood, the too great waste of the body can be supplied by its recreative power so effectually that the debilitating effect is not noticed; but when that power of recreation becomes much diminished, the loss becomes more permanent and apparent. Let the young be admonished lest this useful luxury be used intemperately. Other cases have come under observation, where bathing had been extensively practiced for years, but as age came on, the system was not able longer to bear the excessive exhalations by insensible perspiration which the practice occasioned.

ON AMUSEMENTS

All amusements for recreation should of course be innocent
and free from a tendency to any kind of dissipation. The
periods daily allotted to exercise and relaxation may be more
or less occupied in amusements; but generally there should be,
aside from this, some time occasionally spent exclusively in
simple recreations. There should be occasional hunting parties,
fishing parties, temperance picnics, sleigh rides, and other
pleasure parties and excursions. Occasional plays and games
which have no evil tendency, may be made profitable to
health. Some may think that such recommendations are giving
too great license; but if they are properly chosen and managed,
there can be no harm from them, but great good: they are
recommended not for the sake of the mere amusement they are
adapted to give, but purely for the purpose of recreating and
preserving a healthy state of body and mind; which cannot
always be done without these aids. Those persons especially
who are devoted to constant mental labor, must have resort to
some kind of mental relaxation, or their constitutions will
suffer loss: the mind cannot bear to be kept constantly on the
stretch of exertion; it will soon lose its elasticity and power,
and the body give way.

ON INDULGENCES

Under this head it is intended to speak of things which are
inexpedient and unlawful. While honest and innocent
amusements, used with judgment and temperance, are very
important by way of giving elasticity and strength to the mind

and body, unlawful and intemperate indulgences injure and often ruin both. There are amusements which are innocent and harmless in their nature, that may be used intemperately and unlawfully. Amusements should be used, not as a matter of indulgence, but of actual utility: and while kept under such a rule, all is well; but the moment they shall be used for the simple gratification they give, they are likely to engross too much of time and thought, and lead to ruinous results. But when persons resort to measures for their gratification, which are unlawful when used in any degree, the danger is greatly increased.

Private indulgences claim attention here. Indulgences which belong to married life, when used with moderation, are conducive to health; the married, all other things being equal, enjoy better health and live longer than the single; but when these are allowed in excess, they reduce the vital energies, diminishing the powers of body and mind. All licentiousness, aside from its moral evils and degradation, is destructive to the human system. Many a young man has not only ruined his reputation and moral character, by licentious practices, but has spoiled his constitution for life. He has, early in life, planted in his system the seeds of misery and premature death. One who has early in life given himself to such habits, has unfitted himself for the future enjoyment of domestic happiness. The degradation of his mind, and the vitiation of his appetite, have made him unfit to become the companion of virtue and refinement, and he is very likely to continue the indulgence of his corrupted passions, whatever may be the sacrifice to his moral and physical health.

Self-indulgence is another low-lived, contemptible vice, which has destroyed its thousands and tens of thousands annually, both of males and females. Setting aside a comparison of its sin-fulness, it is doing more injury to society than all other forms of licentiousness put together. Boys, and even girls, of respectable origin, of splendid original talents, have, by this unnatural practice, not only destroyed their physical systems, but have reduced their minds to comparative imbecility, and, in many cases, to complete idiotism. It would seem as though, if one were lost to all sense of moral accountability on this subject, that the idea of making oneself an idiot, to be a walking monument of self-destruction, would be enough, of itself, to deter the most inveterate devotee to his passions, from such habits.

The bodily diseases produced in this way are frequently very formidable, and baffle the most profound skill. Sometimes they appear in the form of spinal affections, which send distress and wretchedness throughout the whole nervous system. Accompanying this, will often be found a morose disposition, dejection of mind, and melancholy. These affections are common to males and females. And added to these, there will not infrequently appear in males, seminal incontinence, wasting away the vital energies; and in females, vaginal discharges, which are no less destructive to health.

MENTAL AFFECTIONS

The sympathy existing between the mind and the body is so great, that when one is affected, both are affected. If a person imagine even that he is sick, he is pretty sure to be sick. If, while in health, he be told, and made to believe, that his countenance indicates illness, in a short time his whole system will become affected. Medicines have sometimes been known to produce their specific effect by a mere dread of taking them. Let the imagination be inspired with confidence that a certain medicine, or coarse of treatment, is going to perform a cure, and the cure is likely to follow. It is on this principle, that simple bread pills have sometimes performed great cures; and on this principle, doubtless, depends, to a very considerable extent, the success of homœopathists.

CHEERFULNESS

This state of mind has much to do with the healthy action of the physical system. A cheerful and happy mind gives a free and easy circulation in the nervous system; it aids in the generation of animal electricity or nervous fluid, which gives support to the vital energies of the whole body. Cheerfulness, by its effect on the nervous system, contributes much toward a healthy and free circulation of the blood. It has to do, indeed, with the formation of the blood, by virtue of its influence on the process of digestion. A cheerful mind, especially during the hour set apart particularly for the first effort of the stomach after a meal, is very important to an easy, thorough digestive process. If the mind be attacked with grief, the food is not digested as well; and consequently the system is not as well nourished. How commonly does leanness of body follow continued grief! Why this? Because grief hinders the process of nutrition. It does it in two ways; it hinders the thorough digestion of the food, so that nutrition cannot as well be extracted from it, and it retards the action of the absorbent vessels themselves, which take up the nutritive part of the food, and convey it into the blood.

Whatever, then, may be an individual's condition or circumstances in life, it will be great economy for him to make himself cheerful and happy. However bitter may be the cause of his grief, let him cultivate a spirit of resignation; however painful may be his condition in life, let him endeavor to be content with such things as he has; however dark his prospects, let him hope for good. While nothing is gained by despondency, much is lost. While cheerfulness helps others to be healthy and happy, it is of great benefit to oneself.

Some have thought that much cheerfulness was contrary to true dignity and Christianity. But this is taking a narrow-minded view of things. It is no more a sin nor a breach of dignity to indulge in real cheerfulness, than it is to take wholesome food. There is a distinction to he made between cheerfulness and levity. While levity may be undignified and unchristian, genuine cheerfulness may be a. part of dignity and Christianity both. Ministers have been sometimes charged with a want of spirituality, because, at some of their social meetings, they indulge in some degree of merriment; but all this is in keeping with nature's law, and is absolutely essential to health. Their situation and calling ordinarily circumscribe them in relation to sources of amusement, and their responsibilities are adapted to induce solemnity of mind; and if this condition could not now and then be relieved, they could scarcely endure it. If we would be benefited by their ministrations, we must give them a chance to live.

MELANCHOLY

This affection of mind has an opposite effect, on the general health, to that of cheerfulness. Melancholy deadens the circulation in the blood vessels and nerves; and also retards the action of the liver. It retards the process of digestion and of nutrition, and tends to dry up the fluids of the whole system.

A state of despondency and melancholy is a frequent accompaniment of deranged digestive organs. It sometimes is found to be both cause and effect. It often causes dyspepsia, and whether it cause it or not, it generally follows it; and then operates both as cause and effect. When melancholy, or a despairing state of mind, once exists, whether as connected with deranged digestive organs, or any other state of ill health, the cure becomes very much more difficult and doubtful; and nothing comparatively can be effected by way of medication, for the benefit of the patient, till something be done for the mental affection. Some method must be had at once to attract the attention of the patient away from himself and his complaints. Hence, in selecting a method of cure, some exercise or. employment must be chosen, which will interest and engage the thoughts, and prevent their being absorbed in himself; and those associated with him must put on the most cheerful aspect.

BENEVOLENCE

Human sympathy is a quality of our natures which the Creator has implanted in us; and whoever cultivates and exercises it, yields to a law of his social character — obeys a law of his nature; and whoever cherishes a due spirit of obedience to any law of his being, is doing that which is promotive of his health. In willing good to others — which necessarily involves all practicable benefactions — there is a pleasant sensation passes over the mind, which also vibrates over the whole body; and this heaven-born vibration of human sympathy and goodwill, gives a glow of health to the whole mental and animal system. Hence, the fact, that in times of the prevalence of pestilential diseases, those who devote themselves to the self-sacrificing effort of nursing and watching the sick and dying, while the victims of the malady are fast falling on their right and left, seldom become a prey to that malignant disease themselves. The great philanthropist, John Howard, could never have endured so long his labors amidst the varied death-damps of prisons and dungeons, and appalling scenes of wretchedness to which he exposed himself, had not the desire and the pleasure of doing good, for the sake of humanity and of God, given to his system unwonted power of resistance to disease and endurance of toil.

He who wills good to his fellow-beings, and. so far as able, gives practical demonstration of his benevolence, is not only relieving the ills of human life in others, but is at the same time contributing largely to his own health of soul and body. The Great Teacher of practical benevolence fully appreciated the personal benefit to be derived from the exercise of a spirit of benevolence, when he said, "It is more blessed to give than to receive." Let those who have never made the experiment, begin at once to yield obedience to this law of their social being, and they will find that in doing so, they will receive their reward.

MALEVOLENCE

This affection of mind is contrary to every law of our social being. Willing evil to our fellow-beings is contrary to the moral law of God, to the law of human brotherhood, and the law of our mental constitution. Whoever indulges this spirit, has sunk out of himself as he was constituted by the hand of his Maker, and become a fit subject for the companionship of demons; where no other feelings than malice and revenge, crimination and recrimination, ever find a dwelling- place. A spirit of revenge for injuries finds a resting- place only in the bosom of fools, who defy the right of the Almighty to declare, "Vengeance is mine; I will repay:" much less will a malicious spirit, without provocation, find a place in his breast, in which any of the milk of human kindness dwells.

Whoever indulges this cold, misanthropic temper of mind, chokes the natural current of his soul; and while that soul is thus constrained, and its social sympathies are becoming dried and withered, the whole physical organization feels its unnatural action, and becomes partaker of its unnatural depravity. This is to be seen in the very countenance. While the face of the benevolent man shines with the luster of moral and physical health, that of the misanthropist is dejected, downcast, and sullen. Why this difference in the physical conformation of the countenance? Because the soul of man gives direction to the action of the whole animal economy; and enstamps its own image upon the outward man. One who is versed at all in reading human character, can easily distinguish a benevolent man from one of malevolent spirit, by his exterior, especially the expression of his face.

OBLIGATIONS TO LAW

PHYSICAL OBLIGATIONS

A man who would enjoy perfect health is obliged to obey physical law; and from this physical obligation he cannot free himself; for if he transgress physical law, he must endure the infliction of a physical penalty. While the violator of human law may escape the punishment due to his crimes, by keeping them out of sight, or by fleeing from the reach of justice, the man who is guilty of violating the laws of his own animal economy, cannot escape with impunity — his sin is sure to find him out. Though he may pass on for a while without arrest, yet sooner or later, he will find himself overtaken, tried before Dame Nature's court, and condemned.

The man, who, by gradual steps, deviates from the path-way of physical law, may seem to pass on uninjured for some length of time, yet, by and by, he will be sure to feel the rod of punishment. The man who disregards dietetic rules, may not at first discover any injury, or if he experience suffering, he may not discover the relation of the cause and the effect, yet the consequences of his unlawful course, will, sooner or later, follow, and he cannot escape. The man who habitually steeps himself in alcoholic liquor, may possibly live to threescore years and ten, and seem to be tolerably well; yet he has made himself liable to fall suddenly dead, in consequence of the unseen fires that have for years been consuming his internal organs. The man who disobeys law in any other way, may not now see that his system is injured, yet when some outward cause of disease may approach him, he is overcome by it, simply because his previous habits have weakened the power of resistance in his constitution.

MORAL OBLIGATIONS

Next to our obligations to God, are our obligations to ourselves. If we are under obligation to treat our Creator right, we are also, next to him, under obligation to treat ourselves right. The second table of the moral law, comprehended in this, "Thou shalt love thy neighbor as thyself," implies the pre-existence of the law of self-love; and the law of self-love involves the obligation of self-protection. What right have we TO abuse, or even to neglect, ourselves? To do that which will injure our constitution or health, is sinful in the sight of Heaven. To transgress physical law is transgressing God's law; for be is as truly the Author of physical law, as he is the Author of the moral law. Whoever, therefore, violates the laws of life and health, sins against God as truly as though he break the ten commandments. Every man is therefore under moral obligation to obey those laws; and whoever dares violate them will find "The way of transgressors is hard."

The moral sense of community is exceedingly obtuse on this subject. With the great majority, appetite is the only law which governs; and in spite of all that can be said, it will probably continue to be so: and those who choose to have it so, must bear the consequences. But some may possibly be induced to examine their obligations and responsibilities in the case. Where is the consistency of being governed by principle instead of appetite, in regard to the demands of the moral law, and yet let appetite rule instead of principle in regard to physical law? for, as before stated, when we violate physical law, we do truly violate moral obligation. Whoever will let appetite govern in one thing, is in a fair way to let it govern in all things. Whoever, through appetite, will allow himself to eat too much or too often, is very likely to give license to all other appetites and passions in proportion to their strength and activity.

PERSONAL OBLIGATIONS

Obedience to the laws of health should he made a matter of individual and personal duty. It is every individual's duty to study the laws of his being and to conform to them. Ignorance or inattention on this subject is sin; and the injurious consequences of such a course make it a case of gradual suicide. The idea that we may do what we please with ourselves, is not only bad policy, and bad economy, but to do so is positively wrong: it is sin against the Author of our being. And when persons knowingly or wantonly expose themselves to disease and death by violating the laws of life and health, instead of calling the result a visitation of Providence, it should be called a suicidal act.

The laboring man who eats quick and works immediately after, is not only pursuing a course of bad economy, but is doing wrong to himself and to his Creator. He is diminishing his power and durability for doing good. When a man of intellectual habits neglects to live in accordance to the laws of mind and body, he pursues not only a bad policy, but secures for himself the punishment due to his criminal conduct. The man who lives unnaturally instead of naturally, who allows his system to come under the influence of stimulating drinks, or unnatural excitants, or narcotic and poisonous drugs, does a material and important wrong to himself, and must expect to give account for his course on the day of final judgment.

The strange abandonment of principle which characterizes this generation in their treatment of themselves, is almost enough to dishearten the most sanguine hopes of reform. Instead of seeking after a true knowledge of themselves — the laws which sustain and govern their own animal existence — and what course of living they ought to adopt to secure for themselves a sound state of health and long life, they foolishly and wickedly inquire, "What shall I eat, and wherewithal shall I enjoy the present hour?."

If we tell the devotee to the alcoholic draft, or the more poisonous and filthy narcotic, tobacco, that his daily potations, or the essences of the deadly weed, are secretly gnawing the tender cords that bind his soul and body together, he heeds us not. He will probably acknowledge the facts in the case, and, at the same time, with most perfect indifference to consequences, and insensibility to personal obligations, will answer, that he chooses rather to enjoy life while he does live, than to prolong life by curtailing present gratification. But what is duty — what is right — in the case?

Have we a right to prefer present gratification to permanent good.? Have we any right to open a vein and let the blood gradually run away because we are delighted with the crimson stream? We have just as much right to do this, as we have to use rum, tobacco, tea, coffee, or any other hurtful agent, for mere gratification, against the highest earthly interests of our own bodily constitutions.

SOCIAL OBLIGATIONS

In addition to our own personal obligations to physical law, we are under additional obligations in consequence of our relations to society. We are under obligations to law for the sake of posterity. Parents, and those who may expect to be parents, are called upon to take care of their health and constitution for the sake of generations to come. If parents are of weakly or diseased constitution, the children must suffer, to more or less extent, the consequences. By the unlawful course of parents in regard to themselves, the children often suffer disease and premature death.

Parents are also under obligation to teach and oblige their children to conform to physical law for their own sakes. The mother who suffers her children to eat irregularly, or violate the laws of their systems in any other way, commits a crime against her offspring, against humanity, and against Heaven, for which God will hold her responsible. She commits a crime against the dearest objects of her affections, the evil consequences of which, time may never be able wholly to remove, and eternity alone reveal to her understanding. How strange and unaccountable, that mothers should love their children so tenderly as to indulge them in what they have occasion to know may injure their constitutions and impair their happiness for life! May many children be delivered from such mothers and from such cruel kindnesses.

The managers and teachers of schools and literary institutions are under obligations to secure such facilities for exercise and regulations in regard to the observance of dietetic law, as are adapted to preserve the health, promote the literary progress, and secure to the world the usefulness of their pupils. And students owe it to the world that they so walk in obedience to law, as to render their existence and advantages a blessing to society.

Professional men cannot disregard the laws of their own health, without infringing upon their obligations to community whom they serve. If their services are required, they are bound to make the most of their ability to meet the demand. The labors of any professional man, engaged in the active business of his calling, whether he be a clergyman, a physician, or a lawyer, make a severe draft upon the nervous system, which will require all the strength that it can possibly command.

Laboring men have a responsibility in this matter. Those of them who employ laborers are bound, not only for their own interests, but for the interests of those who serve them, so to regulate the hours of each day's labor, as to give their men a chance to live, enjoy the blessings of life, and sustain those who may fall into their charge. Those who are employed by others, are under obligation to live in such a manner as to make themselves of service to their employers, and meet the demands of society at large.

All who desire the welfare and improvement of society, are under obligation to endeavor to exert an influence over others on this subject by example and precept. No man can live entirely isolated from his fellow-beings: his influence by word or deed is constantly telling pro or con the well-being of the world. Let Him see to it that it be such, touching this matter, as shall make mankind the better and the happier for his having lived in it. Let him be at least a drop in the bucket of that great wheel which moves the vast machinery of human improvement in its onward course.

APPENDIX

PHILOSOPHY OF HEALTHY REPRODUCTION

THE attention of the public has of late been called to this subject, and a considerable amount of information, in the form of books and lectures, has been disseminated. And certainly that must be a very fastidious taste and a narrow mind which would object to giving to the people, in a judicious style, such a practical knowledge of themselves as is essential to the healthy reproduction of the species. Who should not know enough of the natural origin of human life to perceive his own obligations respecting it, and to be able to see in what way he is liable to be a curse, or in what way a blessing, to posterity?

All information, however, given on this subject for mere mercenary purposes, or to pamper an idle and vicious curiosity, should be most sternly repudiated. Nor is it best, even for laudable intentions, to go further into detail on these delicate matters, than is really necessary for the practical purposes of life. But so far as these do require information to be given, all whimpering delicacy and superfluous niceness should be looked out of countenance by the firm and steadfast eye of common sense. Let every individual so study himself and know himself, as to be able in this matter to discharge his responsibilities to humanity and to God.

This consists in the germinating principle; which contains probably the entire infinitesimal rudiment of the future being. This germ, when examined by the aid of the microscope, is found to contain animalcule Their form bears a striking resemblance to the human brain and spinal column. Those which proceed from a robust constitution manifest great vital energy; while those from a constitution of an opposite kind exhibit an opposite character. In conjunction with its appropriate and tributary maternal element, this germ ultimately becomes developed into perfectly organized vitality.

This germinating principle has its origin unquestionably in the brain and nervous system; particularly that portion of the brain called cerebellum. To this part belongs the organ of emotiveness; on the existence of which the propagation of the species depends. On the healthy development and action of this organ, under the balancing and regulating power of intellect and moral sentiment, together with the vital qualities of a sound physical system, depend, in a very large degree, the physical and mental force which shall belong to the future offspring.

On the healthy condition of the bodily system depends the vital energy of the germinating principle. Numerous experiments of learned physiologists show this statement to be correct. The legitimate conclusion, therefore, must inevitably be, that the innate constitution of the offspring must bear an immediate and necessary relation to the vital power of that system from which the germ proceeds.

In proof that the brain and nerves have a direct and positive agency in this matter, it is a well attested fact, that in all cases of excess — a condition most injurious to the parent and the offspring — there is found a complaint of a peculiar and enervating sensation in the head, especially in the region of the cerebellum, accompanied with a degree of general nervous prostration. In some instances there will be a periodical or protracted head-ache, which can only be removed when the cause ceases to be, and the immediate effects have passed away. That the quality of the paternal system, especially the brain and nerves, determines the character of the offspring, is, therefore, a tangible matter of fact.

PATERNAL RESPONSIBILITY

In view of these facts, just adduced, the responsibilities which fall on those who are now liable, or may at some future period become liable, to be fathers, are incalculable. That man who practically disregards his obligations touching this matter, is not fit for the society of intelligent beings. While he lives as he lists, following out his depraved and self-created appetites, regardless of his obligations to himself, his generation, and his God, he is only fit to herd among swine and grovel in the mire of his own sensuality. We see that the rudiment of the future being is of paternal origin, and that the quality of constitution possessed by the parent determines in a great degree the character of that future being. Hence the conclusion is legitimate, that inattention to such responsibilities is in a high degree reprehensible.

Any departure from strict obedience to nature's laws tends to weaken the system. And any process which, in any degree, produces this result, proportionably disables an individual for meeting his obligations to his race. That man who uses alcoholic liquors, is steeping his brain and nerves in the poisonous cup. He is taking one of the most deadly enemies to human life into the very citadel of his being. His brain, from whence the germ of a future being proceeds, is steaming and fuming by the alcoholic fires which he has there kindled. Can this man suppose that he can take his daily, or even occasional dram, and his children escape the consequences? Ay, they cannot escape. As a general rule — which may have exceptions — there will be found unusual physical or moral defects; and perhaps both.

A case in proof is at hand: a father of nine children became by degrees a confirmed drunkard. When first married, and until after his fourth child was born, he remained temperate; but being unfortunate in business, he suddenly became, and continued, addicted to his cups; during which time his other five children were born. One of these was convicted of robbery, and served an apprenticeship in the state prison; another of theft; another of larceny; another became a drunkard; the fifth was an idiot. The mother of all these was an excellent woman, and his first four children were intelligent and upright. These facts are not alone; many are there of a similar character which testify to the same general truth.

That man who chews and smokes his tobacco, is the individual to be addressed on this subject. He is doing that to himself which should be called gradual suicide; and that for his future offspring which should be denominated manslaughter. It is to him that truth would direct her long and pointed finger, saying, "Thou art the man." His brain and nerves are tinctured with that foul and loathsome thing, which none else will ever eat except the miserable tobacco worm, and the rock goat of Africa, whose effluvia none but himself can endure. He is daily taking into his system an amount perhaps of the real essence of that wretched poison sufficient, when given to those who are unaccustomed to its use, to destroy at once the lives of half a dozen men. His nervous susceptibilities to its immediate effects are blunted; but the genuine poison, which, under other circumstances, would kill him, and many others with him, is nevertheless lodged daily in his system, and must sooner or later cause him to pay the penalty of violated law.

And where principally has this poison lodged itself? On the brain and nerves. It is through this medium making gradual inroads upon his own physical and mental systems, and those of his immediate posterity. His brain, which is to give origin to other beings, is saturated with the poison. A poison, too, which affects not only his brain and nerves, but every gland, every membrane, and every tissue of his body. His children cannot escape being sharers of its hurtful agency. In view of this undeniable fact, will our young men, for fashion's sake, or for a depraved, unnatural appetite's sake, continue this wicked gratification? Will they, in spite of consequences, and in defiance of solemn obligation, go on, puffing their cigars or chewing the deadly weed? Do they lack for moral courage to face and defend themselves against that created, depraved and infernal appetite? Are they beyond the reach of recovery — drawn down the current of an enslaving and overpowering propensity? Do they give it up? or has tobacco so deadened their moral sensibilities — which it is capable of doing — that they can look upon this whole subject with a dogged indifference?

People are apt to think that because a certain habit — which they perhaps in theory admit to be bad — does not destroy life, or immediately make them invalids, they are getting no harm, and are under no need or obligation to change their course. They judge of their obligations to physical law as they do of their obligations to moral law; that because judgment against an evil-doer is not executed speedily, they may sin on with impunity. But punishment for violated physical law will sooner or later come; and if they who offend could bear the rod alone, their crime against nature's government would seem to be of less consequence; but when we know that their innocent offspring must bear a part of the punishment due to their parents, their offense seems to swell to a tenfold magnitude.

Tobacco is one of the most deadly narcotics found upon the list of poisons. A very few drops of its condensed properties will destroy life. It is sometimes used as a medicine, though rarely, in extreme cases, where nothing else will meet the indications in the case. When used, it is generally given by injection, in cases of lock-jaw, convulsions, and so on; but is never given by those who understand its properties, but with the utmost caution: a little imprudence might prove fatal. It should never be used as a medicine except by a judicious physician, even by external application; for so powerful are its poisonous qualities that a small quantity, laid upon the skin, may prove fatal by mere absorption. If any doubt can be indulged in regard to its power, let any one who has never used it chew a small piece, and the genuine power of the article will soon manifest itself. And though the habitual use of it stupefies the nervous susceptibilities, yet the real power of the article is daily absorbed into the system, and is doing by degrees, and perhaps by imperceptible progress, its deadly work. And now returns the momentous question, in view of all the consequences, shall this demon-idol be longer worshipped, or trodden under foot?

All forms of licentiousness are destructive; not only to those who indulge it, but those who may have the sad misfortune to inherit its poisonous fruits. This vice prostrates the whole nervous system, and is destructive to that principle which becomes the origin of life. If those who have ruined their constitutions by habits of this kind should ever become fathers, their children will probably give them sufficient proof that such a paternal relationship is never to be coveted. Another form of licentiousness, no less ruinous to posterity, is, self-indulgence. This secret vice is all but ruining the whole race. It often begins very early in life, and continues till its work of destruction — if it has not utterly annihilated the reproductive power — has so enfeebled it as to render marriage inexpedient and even improper.

Any coarse of conduct or habit of living which tends to lower the standard of nervous strength, or to vitiate the fluids of the system, is deleterious to the constitution of the offspring. Every one who ever expects to become a parent, should obey his own physical laws in all things, not merely for himself, but for the sake of his immediate generation.

Mental health, also, is essential to healthy reproduction. Great mental exertion and application — that application which tends, even temporarily, to diminish the mental force, is injurious for the time being to the reproductive power. This may account for the fact — in part at least — that great men seldom leave sons who are able to fill the places of their fathers. The talent of the child may not so much depend upon the degree of talent possessed by the parent, as upon the good condition of his physical, mental, and moral systems. A healthy physical system, with well- balanced brain and nerves, and a well-cultivated moral and intellectual character, make up, then, the great leading qualifications to meet our responsibilities touching this subject.

There is another idea connected with this subject which may be important. There should he in all cases, particularly in men of studious habits, a sufficiency of mental exhilaration, as well as bodily exercise, to maintain an equilibrium of nervous circulation. The clerical profession are in special need of care touching this matter. Their calling involves the general idea, especially in the mind of a scrutinizing community, of great and uniform sedateness of deportment. Hence, partly from the nature of their calling, and partly from the expectations of the people, they are accustomed to suppress that natural buoyancy of spirit, and that letting off of the electricity of mirthfulness, which are common to all persons, and which, for health's sake, should, in some proper way, find opportunity to vent itself.

This suppression of nature's promptings must cause a kind of continual or occasional desire for mirth, which is kept pent up in the cloisters of the soul. It is the same feeling in kind which the boy felt, and could not suppress, when he whistled aloud during the hours of school. Being asked, "Did you whistle, John?" he promptly answered in the negative. "George, did not John whistle?" "Yes, sir." "John, how is that — did you not whistle?" "No, sir — it whistled itself." This same kind of would-if-it-could feeling must inevitably exist within those who are comparatively deprived of the privilege of sufficient mental recreation. This may very philosophically account for that proverbial saying, which certainly has some foundation in fact, that the sons of clergymen are the greatest rogues. They have this same would-if-it-could disposition inborn in their mental constitutions.

THE MATERNAL PRINCIPLE OF REPRODUCTION

This consists in what is called the ovum, or egg, which bears a close resemblance in character to that of the oviparous or egg-bearing animals. This is the natural element for the reception of the primary principle or germ which is of paternal origin. It is located, not in the interior, as may generally be supposed, but is on the exterior, upper, and lateral part of the uterus, or womb. The whole course of the reproductive process is, in all its essential features, analogous to that of oviparous reproduction. Soon after the reproductive process is commenced, the ovum changes its location from the exterior to the interior of the uterus, where it undergoes a full fetal development. The uterine system is concerned in the nutrition and perfection of the paternal rudiment of the future being; and great care should be taken that nothing, at any stage of early life, shall transpire to derange its functionary powers, and disable it for the purposes for which it was originally designed.

This system is liable to derangements of various kinds. One is displacement. This may be brought about by severe lifting; jumping and striking hard upon the feet; long protracted standing; severe exercise in jumping rope; severe exercise in dancing; tight lacing; and other causes. Any cause, too, which tends to weaken the general system will greatly promote this derangement. Irregularities of periodical habit often become matters of serious moment. Where daughters have been brought up under proper physical training — if their discipline in respect to diet, open air, exercise, and other things, has been what they should be — there will be little difficulty of this kind. But if parents have been guilty of neglecting these obligations, have brought up their daughters too delicately, have not given sufficient attention to the development of their physical powers, or have allowed them to have irregular habits of diet, by which their digestive apparatus has become disordered, serious results may follow. If they have not given them precautions against such causes as sudden colds, exposure of the feet by thin shoes, long-continued cold feet, tight lacing, costive bowels, and other hurtful influences, they may find occasion for repentance when it is too late to make amends.

There is great sympathy between the female mind and her own reproductive system. The offspring, while in its fetal state, receives an imprint from the maternal mind, which, though it may afterward be modified, can never be eradicated. It there receives a mental and moral mould, the great outlines of which can never be obliterated. We go into a family of children, and find some very different traits of character. Trace the history of these different children back to their fetal state, and the influences to which they were then exposed by the immediate operations of the mother's mind, and the causes of these differences will then appear. While the paternal character gives the great features, the immediate operations of maternal influences give the smaller peculiarities.

This sympathy is also manifested in the effects of sudden emotions and particular appetites. Deformities of physical structure are not infrequently produced by a sudden impression being made on the mother's mind by the unexpected appearance of some frightful or disagreeable object. A case which has come under the observation of the writer, was of this sort. The mother, during her pregnancy — somewhere about the sixth month — indulged a great desire for partridge-meat. The husband went in search for the fowl, but rinding none, killed a ground-squirrel, and brought it home. She saw him at a distance, thought the partridge was coming, and prepared her cooking apparatus for its reception. She saw no more of her husband till he, with astonishing imprudence, threw the dead animal at her feet. She was shocked at the sight, and sadly disappointed. When the child was born, it presented, in a striking manner, the features of the dead squirrel, as it laid prostrate before her. The arms could never be raised above an angle of forty-five degrees from the body. The hands resembled the animal's claws; the elbow and knee joints were almost immovable, and bent in the opposite way from the natural direction. He lived to ripe manhood, but with the same degree of malformation and disability. Many illustrations of this kind might be adduced, together with cases of mothers' marks, in proof of the great sympathy between the maternal reproductive system and the maternal mind.

MATERNAL EESPONSIBILITY

In anticipation of coming responsibilities, every young woman is bound to look well to herself. She can but know that the grand arrangement of nature is that she shall become a mother. Let her also know that her own state of constitution will in a great degree be the type of that of her future offspring. The talent, the moral tone, and the physical health of that offspring will very much depend on her. Let her weigh this matter well, and prepare herself to meet approaching obligations. Let her be prepared to give the right stamp of character to that living immortal being that may hereafter be committed to her charge.

Let her look well to her physical system. Let her diet and exercise be such as to secure a sound and well- balanced nervous system. Let her strenuously and scrupulously avoid all stimulating drinks and condiments which conflict with nature's laws, and do great mischief to the brain and nerves. Let her live naturally, and not artificially. Let her avocations and exercise be such as will give expansion and strength to her whole muscular system. Let her take special pains to expand her chest, that her breathing apparatus may be free in the exercise of its vital functions; for without a full chest, she may plant the seeds of consumption in the constitution of her offspring before its birth.

Let her look well to the character of her own moral constitution. Let her choose those dietetic habits which favor moral culture; and which will tend to give a preponderance to the moral sentiment over the animal system. For the sake of her posterity, if for no other purpose, let her make herself an intellectual being; Let her not live for the mere purpose of mercenary and selfish gratifications, but for God and humanity. Let her not live to eat, and drink, and sleep, but to answer the great purposes of her being.

Let her look well to the character of him who may become her matrimonial associate. Is he an intellectual being, or a mere animal? He should have a good physical system, but has he a soul? Is he a sensual being, living for no other purpose than to fill up the measure of his appetites and passions? Has he corrupted his body and soul by dissolute habits? Are his habits of life adapted to secure to him a sound physical system? for if his course of life is weakening and vitiating his bodily nature, a degree of moral imbecility will be likely to follow in its wake. Is he cultivating a sound nervous system, or is he wantonly pursuing a course that is diminishing the natural energy of his brain and nerves, which will unfit him to meet his responsibility to his posterity?

Let her examine well his temperance habits. Does he appreciate the cause of temperance? if not, there is prima facie evidence, in these days of light, of a laxness of moral principle which endangers moral rectitude. Is he a young man of total abstinence habits? or does he now and then take a pleasurable draft? If so, he is dealing with that which may, sooner or later, "bite like a serpent and sting like an adder." Trust him not. He is gradually stepping forward and onward in that path which has conducted millions to ruin. Think of the unmeasured woes of the drunkard's family; then stand aloof and be excused from such a destiny. Is the number of the pure small? then prefer single blessedness to double misery. Nay; let the young men of this generation know that they must quit their occasional drams, or go forever wifeless. Let them know that the young women of this generation cannot consent to share with them so fearful a responsibility as that of having a family of children whose only inheritance must be the hereditary taint of a drunken father.

Let her see whether there is any other hurtful habit of which he is the slave. If he he free from the corrupting and debasing power of alcohol, is he free from that slower, surer, and more deadly poison, tobacco? Let every young lady who sets any value upon herself, look well to this matter. When she sees a young man so lacking in the essential qualities of a gentleman that he needs a cigar to finish him, let her be determined that she will prefer the acquaintance of those who do not require this appendage. And let her never suffer herself to be courted by one of corrupted breath and TOBAOCONIZED BRAIN. Let her never marry one whose habits will ever annoy her, and whose system is under a poison that is enervating the vital and moral energies of his whole nervous constitution, and that will affect her posterity.

Will any one say this is a matter of fancy and not of fact? How comes it that the general idea that the physical condition of parents has a bearing upon the physical character of children, is universally admitted, and yet there are no individual instances in which it is true? The truth is that there are individual instances the world over, and everywhere; but nobody seems to realize it; yet in every case where either of the parents' habits are contrary to physical law, they are doing an injury which. will be more or less felt in the generation following them.

Let every young woman and every young man bring

common sense and reason to hear upon this great and momentous subject. Let them so take care of themselves as to be prepared for the sober realities of life. Let them so fulfill their responsibilities, as that, when years shall have passed away, and their family circle is gathered around them, they may not have cause to look back with sorrow upon the past, and with fearful forebodings toward the future. Let them be so careful in the selection of connubial associates, that they may prove a mutual comfort to each other, and a blessing to the generations which follow them.

Let them beforehand count the cost of indulgence in intemperate appetites and sensual dispositions, which must inevitably tend to en-stamp upon their offspring grossness of moral depravity. Let them not in this way make themselves responsible for the evil conduct of their children, which may bring their gray hairs with sorrow to the grave. But let them, by their physical, moral, and intellectual culture of themselves, be prepared to bring into existence a class of beings whose physical, moral, and intellectual character shall enable them to enjoy life, be an ornament to society, and a blessing to the world.

CONCLUSION

THE preceding pages were written with the sincere hope of doing good to humanity. There is no subject belonging to this life more important than the true science of health. The standard of general health is constantly declining from generation to generation, and the whole cause may be found in the habits of the people. The grand question for the reader is, will he follow every suggestion in this little work, which commends itself to his good sense, endeavoring to raise the standard of strength in his own system, and be prepared to transmit health and soundness to his posterity? Will he live according to the principles of physiological law, and reap the benefits to himself and his progeny? or will he make a god of his belly, suffer the penalty of violated law, and bring disease and premature death on himself and those that follow him?

What shall be said of him who will go on in known hurtful indulgences — feeding unnatural appetites, or crowding his natural ones by unnatural burdens? Shall he be reckoned among intelligent beings — beings endowed with a soul? Inspiration calls that man a fool who seeks only worldly good, and neglects his higher destiny. And is a man any less a fool who knows no higher rule of life than the mere gratification of a depraved appetite; indulgence which hazards health and life, and lowers the standard of his intellectual and moral being? In doing this he puts himself on a level with the soulless brute! Some even put themselves far below the brute! They cherish appetites so low, and vulgar, and unnatural, that brutes will not stoop to be their associates. Brutes will not sip the drunkard's drink; they will not chew the tobacco eater's cud.

How would the ox, or the horse, the dog, or even the muddy swine, degrade his nature, were he to use tobacco — that deadly thing which is working greater devastations to this generation than even alcohol itself! What would a man think to find his horse eating the poisonous stuff? Would he not be alarmed for its effects on his strength and durability? — for every one of much intelligence knows it to be injurious to animal life. Let that same man ask himself whether his own body is worth less than that of his beast; and inasmuch as he has a higher nature, let it be saved from the benumbing influence of the deadly weed. If intelligent beings would live as lawfully as the brute creation, they would as seldom be affected with disease. Will they be lower than the brutes?

Let him who was made to be a man, BE A MAN; or, if not, let him down on all four, and no longer pretend to be what he is not. If he is endowed with reason, let him govern himself; let him study to understand, and resolve to obey the laws of his being, which are the LAWS OF GOD. Let each one resolve to do what he can to turn back the mighty current of physical and moral declension, which now threatens the extinction of the noble qualities of human nature. Let him not live, like the beasts that perish, to gratify his lower nature; let him improve his higher being, LIVE FOR GOD AND HUMANITY.

www.ingramcontent.com/pod-product-compliance
Lightning Source LLC
Chambersburg PA
CBHW051725170526
45167CB00002B/809